# 400 Self Assessment Picture Tests in Clinical Medicine

# 400
# Self Assessment
# Picture Tests in
# Clinical Medicine

**Year Book Medical Publishers, Inc.**

35 E. Wacker Drive—Chicago

©Wolfe Medical Publications Limited 1984

This book is copyrighted in England and may not be
reproduced by any means in whole or part.
Distributed in North America and Canada by
Year Book Medical Publishers, Inc.
by arrangement with Wolfe Medical Publications Ltd.

Library of Congress Cataloging in Publication Data

400 self-assessment picture tests in clinical medicine.

1. Diagnosis—Atlases.   2. Diagnosis—Examinations,
questions, etc.   I. Year Book Medical Publishers.
II. Title: Four hundred self-assessment picture tests
in clinical medicine. [DNLM: 1. Diagnosis—Atlases.
2. Diagnosis—Problems. WB 18 Z99]
RC71.3.A17   1984     616.07'5      83-26120
International Standard Book Number: ISBN 0-8151-9403-X

Printed by Royal Smeets Offset b.v., Weert, Netherlands

# Preface

The Color Atlas series, co-published by Year Book Medical Publishers (Chicago) and Wolfe Medical Publications Ltd. (London) represents a source of over 100 medicine specialty atlases featuring well over 40,000 diagnostic color pictures of superior quality. **400 Self-Assessment Picture Tests in Clinical Medicine** draws from nearly 40 titles from the Color Atlas series.

The authors of the atlases listed on the following page chose favorite illustrations depicting diagnostic dilemmas from their own books. Then each author devised questions about his pictures designed to sharpen the diagnostic skills of clinicians at all levels of experience and sophistication.

The questions accompanying these illustrations vary enormously, deliberately so. Some are apparently easy but actually present interesting problems in differential diagnosis. Others appear difficult in some respects but have very straightforward answers. Still others are a mixture of qualities designed to elicit diverse views about the condition.

All 400 picture tests are uniformly presented. Each test is illustrated by a color photograph, which is unidentified but is captioned with a question indirectly suggestive of the diagnostic pathway. Answers appear on separate pages, beginning on page 249.

The book source for each illustration is listed with each answer. Listing the books with the corresponding pictures and questions might make answering the questions easier, which is not the intention of the book!

We hope clinicians of all sorts will benefit from considering the many facets suggested by the pictures presented here, and that they will be reminded what a powerful diagnostic tool their eyes can and must be.

# Acknowledgements

*The pictures, questions and answers in this book have kindly been provided by the following authors of many of the Color Atlas Series. The titles are listed on page 7.*

Dr. Michael Baraitser
Mr. Michael A. Bedford
Dr. A. Besson
Dr. A. Bloom
Uta Boundy
Dr. A. C. Boyle
Professor J. C. Brocklehurst
Mr. T. R. Bull
Dr. C. D. Calnan
Dr. R. A. Chole
Mr. W. Bruce Conolly
Dr. M. B. L. Craigmyle
Dr. D. R. Davies
Dr. Martha Dynski-Klein
Dr. R. T. D. Emond
Dr. David Evered
Dr. Geoffrey Farrer-Brown
Mr. R. Fawkes
Professor Herbert M. Gilles
Mr. James Gow
Dr. Raymond Greene
Dr. W. Guthrie
Professor Reginald Hall
Mr. R. Haskell
Dr. S. M. Herber
Dr. John Ireland
Dr. D. Geraint James
Dr. A. Kamal

Mr. L. W. Kay
Professor Lipmann Kessel
Dr. Erna E. Kritzinger
Dr. G. M. Levene
Mr. R. W. Lloyd-Davies
Dr. Donald S. McLaren
Professor R. D. G. Milner
Dr. Malcolm Parsons
Dr. Victor Parsons
Professor Wallace Peters
Professor Montague Ruben
Professor F. Saegesser
Dame Professor Sheila Sherlock
Professor Lewis Spitz
Dr. G. M. Steiner
Dr. Peter R. Studdy
Dr. John A. Summerfield
Professor V. R. Tindall
Dr. W. R. Tyldesley
Mr. William F. Walker
Dr. George Williams
Mr. J. G. P. Williams
Dr. Robin M. Winter
Dr. Anthony Wisdom
Dr. Barry E. Wright
Professor R. B. Zachary
Dr. M. Zatouroff

All the illustrations used in this book have appeared in the following color Atlases. The code in bold type following each title is repeated by the side of the answer and thus the source of the illustration may readily be identified. Example **ld** — illustration comes from **Color Atlas of Liver Disease.**

Color Atlas of Bone Diseases **bd**
Color Atlas of Cardiac Pathology **cpa**
Color Atlas of Chest Trauma **chtr**
Color Atlas of Clinical Genetics **clge**
Color Atlas of Clinical Gynecology **clgy**
Color Atlas of Clinical Neurology **cln**
Color Atlas of Clinical Orthopaedics **clo**
Color Atlas of Contact Lenses **col**
Color Atlas of Dermatology **dy**
Color Atlas of Diabetes **di**
Color Atlas of Ear Disease **ed**
Color Atlas of Endocrinology **end**
Color Atlas of ENT Diagnosis **ent**
Color Atlas of the Eye and Systemic Disease **esd**
Color Atlas of General Surgical Diagnosis **gsd**
Color Atlas of Geriatric Medicine **gem**
Color Atlas of Hand Conditions **hc**
Color Atlas of Histology **hi**
Color Atlas of Infectious Diseases **ind**

Color Atlas of Injury in Sport **is**
Color Atlas of Liver Disease **ld**
Color Atlas of the Newborn **nb**
Color Atlas of Nutritional Disorders **nd**
Color Atlas of Ophthalmological Diagnosis **od**
Color Atlas of Oral Medicine **om**
Color Atlas of Oro-facial Diseases **ofd**
Color Atlas of Pediatrics **pd**
Color Atlas of Pediatric Surgical Diagnosis **psd**
Color Atlas of Peripheral Vascular Diseases **pvd**
Color Atlas of Physical Signs in General Medicine **psgm**
Color Atlas of Renal Diseases **rd**
Color Atlas of Respiratory Diseases **resd**
Color Atlas of Rheumatology **rh**
Color Atlas of Surgical Pathology **sp**
Color Atlas of Tropical Medicine and Parasitology **tmp**
Color Atlas of Urology **ur**
Color Atlas of Venereology **ve**

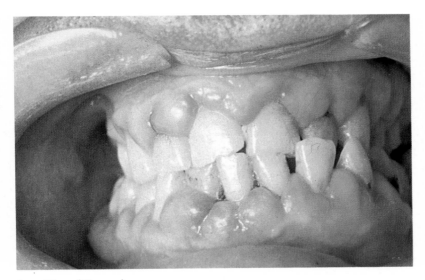

**1.** Firm (fibrous) enlargement of the gums may be due to which drugs?

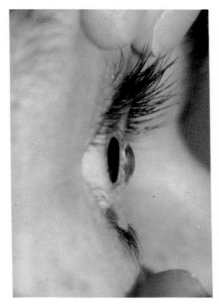

**2.** What is the diagnosis of this conical cornea?

9

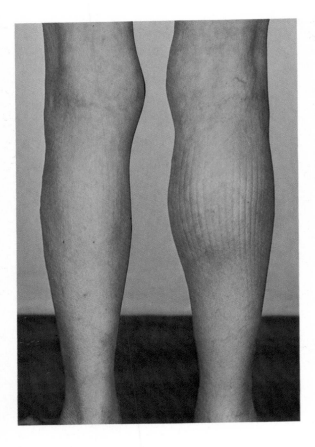

**3.** A painful cystic swelling in right calf and a painful right knee joint suggests the patient could be suffering from which of the following?

a) Osteomyelitis
b) Deep vein thrombosis
c) Rheumatoid arthritis
d) Ruptured muscle
e) Rabdomyosarcoma

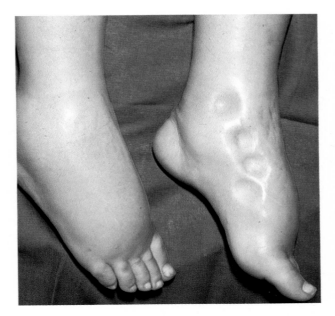

**4.** Gross pitting oedema in a woman who has had diabetes for 20 years. What is the likely cause?

**5.** This object appeared under the conjunctiva of a man returning from long residence in Nigeria. What is it?

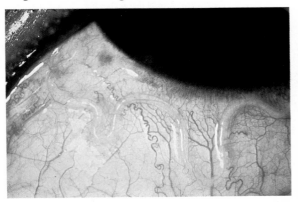

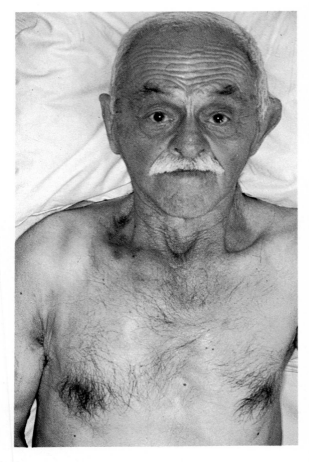

**6.** Does this show the typical appearance of a patient who:

    a) is oppositional as a result of schizophrenia?

    b) is on the point of vomiting?

    c) could have sustained chest injury?

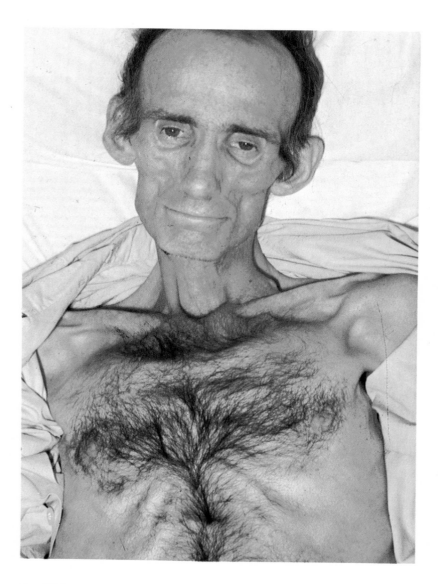

**7.** This man presented with indigestion. What physical sign can you see which suggests the possible diagnosis?

**8.** A meat inspector found these flat objects in the bile ducts of a slaughtered sheep. What are they and are they infectious to man?

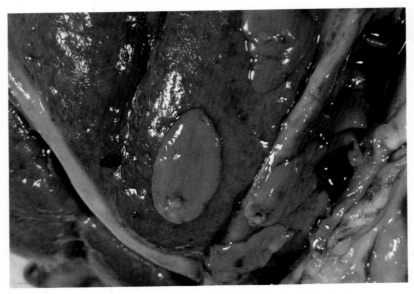

**9.** Rheumatoid nodules on the forearm. What is their prognostic significance?

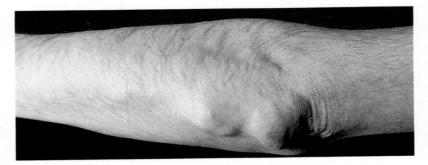

**10.** The patient complains of blurred vision. What is the diagnosis and how would you manage it?

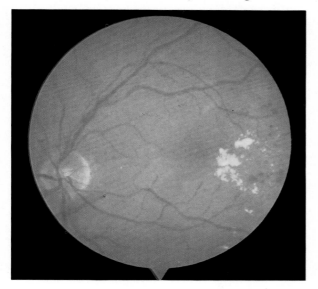

**11.** Magenta coloured painful tongue is common in what vitamin deficiency?

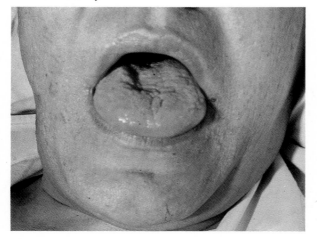

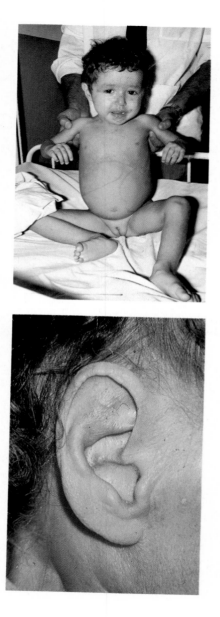

**12.** This Maltese child had chronic fever, anaemia, massive splenomegaly and hepatomegaly. What is the likely diagnosis?

**13.** What is the name of this condition?

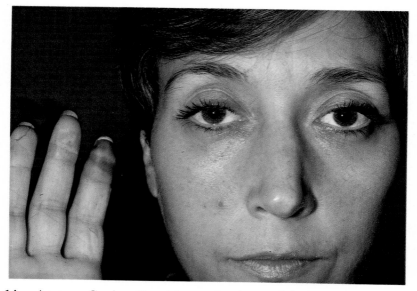

**14.** A young Cook suffered from migraine, and during a severe winter she presented with the physical signs seen in the photograph. What is wrong with her finger? Is this a burn or ischaemic change? Why does the right eyelid droop? What are the physical signs and how can you relate these two together to arrive at a cause?

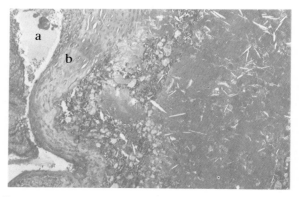

**15.** a) Name the disease   b) List the pathological features shown

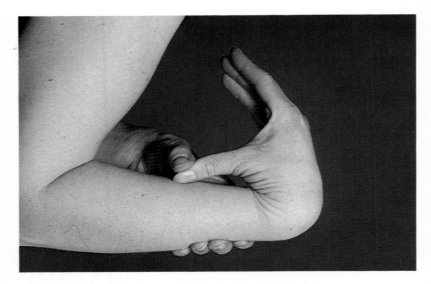

**16.** What is this condition called? What may be its long term consequence?

**17.** a) What two minor abnormalities are seen in this hand?
b) What is the frequency of these in the general population?
c) Of what chromosomal syndrome is this appearance most characteristic?

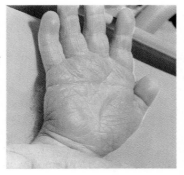

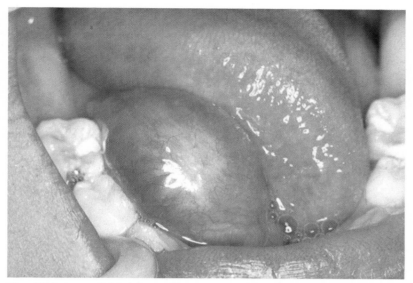

**18.** This is a soft bluish swelling on one side of the floor of the mouth in a child aged 4 — what is the diagnosis?

**19.** Right hand with contracted wrist, thumb and fingers. What has caused these deformities?

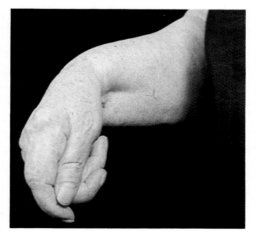

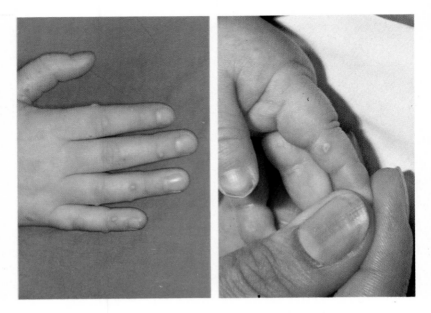

**20.** A child has a mild feverish illness accompanied by a sparse rash on its hands.

a) Would you expect to find lesions elsewhere?
b) Is it infectious?
c) What is the cause?

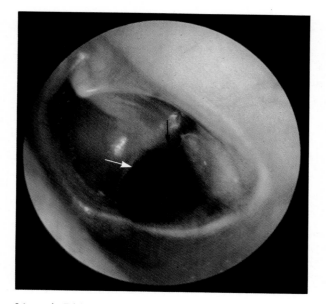

**21.** a) This patient came in complaining of a slight hearing loss and tinnitus. What is your interpretation of the otoscopic finding indicated by the arrows?

b) Is surgical intervention indicated?

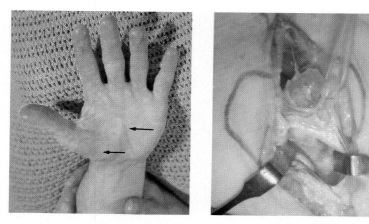

22. **History:** This 35-year-old surgeon presented with a tender swelling at the base of his thenar eminence.
**Examination:** Tender translucent swelling, thenar muscle weakness and wasting.
What is the diagnosis and treatment?

23. a) Describe what you see.
b) Suggest a diagnosis.
c) Itemise helpful investigations.
d) What investigation is contraindicated?
e) What is the treatment?

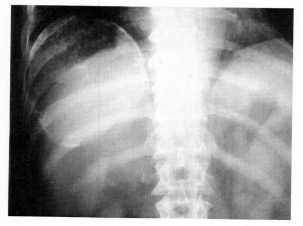

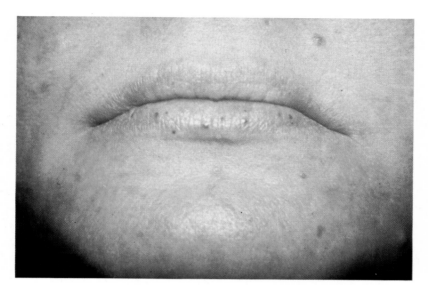

**24.** This abnormality of the lips (also mouth and nose) is an instantly recognisable cause of anaemia due to recent gastro-intestinal haemorrhage — name the syndrome?

**25.** Why is the pupil area opaque in this three months old baby?

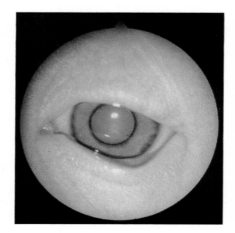

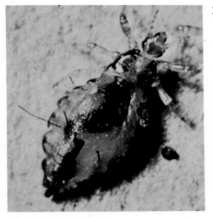

**26.** What is this insect? Can it carry any diseases to man?

**27.** The patient complains of a sore swollen eyelid of several days duration.
What is the condition and how would you manage it?

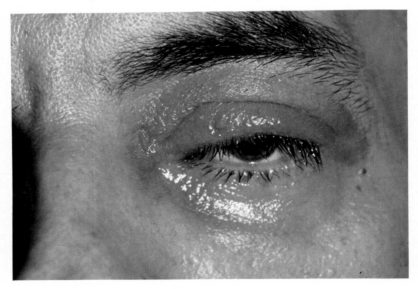

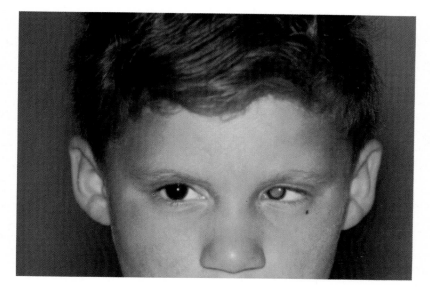

**28.** What is the condition? What could be the underlying cause in this case? What are the commonest causes of this problem and how would you manage them?

**29.** a) What is the diagnosis?
b) Name one important complication?
c) Name the commonest eye sign?
d) What are the risks to offspring?

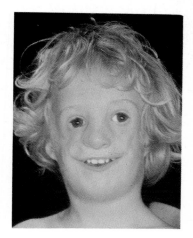

**30.** A patient from the Indian sub-continent presents with hypopigmented patches on the skin. What diagnosis should be excluded?

**31.** a) This patient is diabetic. What is this lesion?
b) What is its underlying cause?
c) Might this affect treatment of the diabetes?

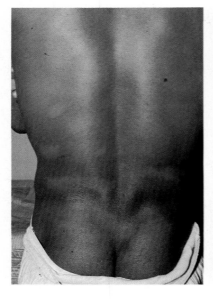

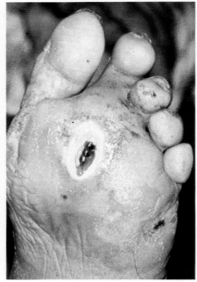

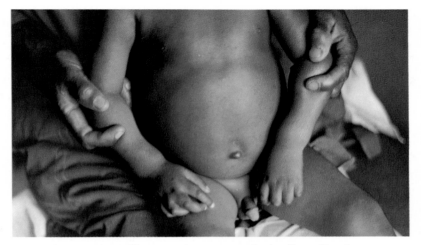

**32.** Abnormal swellings can be seen on the bodies of both
patients — what nutritional abnormality have they in
common and what is the swelling due to?

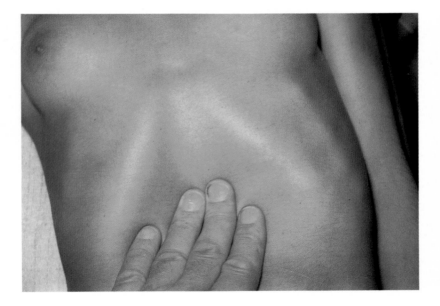

**33.** A well-nourished six-month-old child suddenly develops colicky abdominal pain, vomits and produces blood and mucus in the stool. What is the lesion demonstrated at surgery? What alternative method of treatment is available?

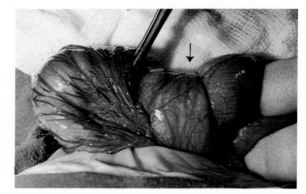

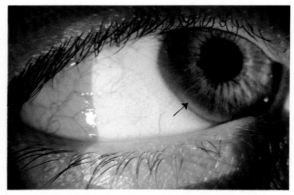

**34.** A patient with renal calculi, back pain and polyuria is found to have an abnormality of the cornea which helped in the diagnosis. The most likely cause of this band was:

a) Hyperlipidaemia
b) Hypercalcaemia
c) Hyperphosphataemia
d) Oxalosis
e) Sarcoidosis

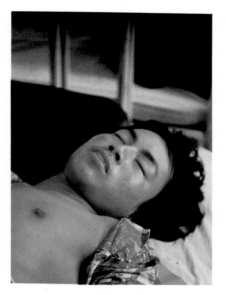

**35.** This patient had just returned from Thailand and presented with fever and coma. What is the diagnosis?

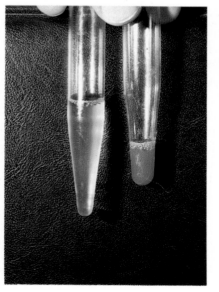

**36.** A patient complained of passing blood in the urine. He had recently been on a business trip in West Africa and had swum in a river. What is the diagnosis?

**37.** This man complained that his shirt got wet, because of a discharge from the nipples. What is this? He was a heavy smoker. Does this suggest a cause?

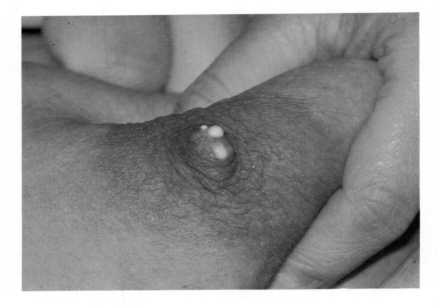

**38.** Acute iritis. In which two rheumatic conditions does this most commonly occur?

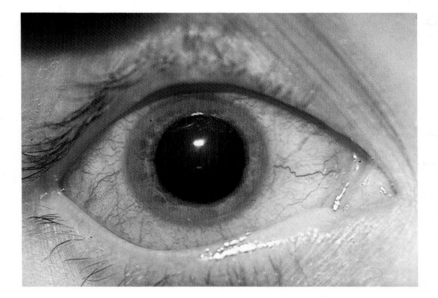

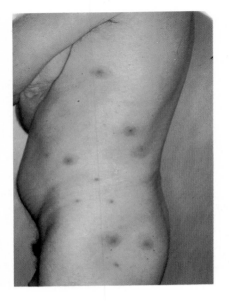

**39.** This man complained of painful "boils" following a stay in West Africa. What is the cause of these lesions?

**40.** What is the diagnosis?

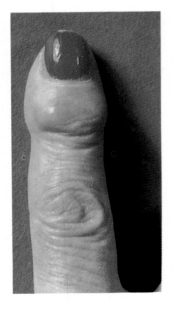

**41.** The terminal phalanges are swollen and the patient complains of pains in the limbs. What does the X-ray show? What investigation would you perform?

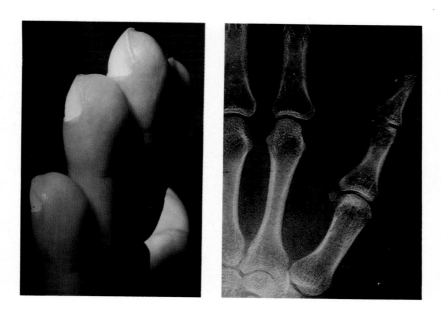

**42.** The entire left shoulder of this elderly patient is occupied by a huge fluctuant mass incorporating the subacromial bursa and the shoulder joint.

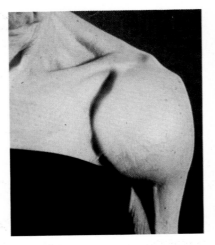

**43.** What is the diagnosis?

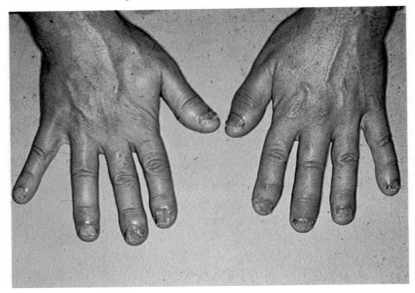

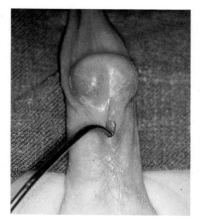

**44.** What is this anomaly of the penis? Of what do the parents most frequently complain? When should treatment be advised?

**45.** What is the abnormality of this well formed infant?

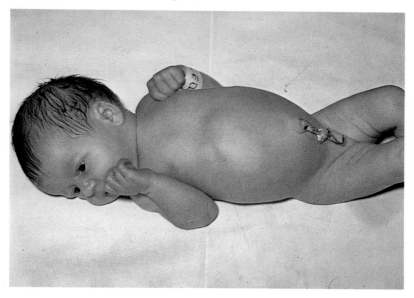

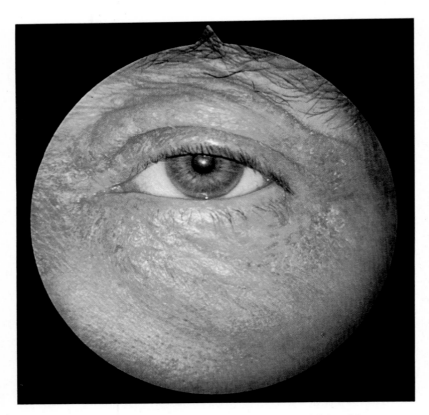

**46.** The patient complains of a sore, itchy eye and lids with perhaps a history of the use of eye drops. What is the condition?

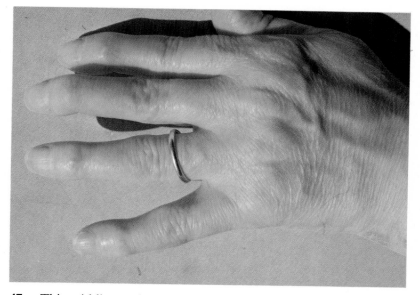

**47.** This middle aged woman complains of swelling of the fingers, limited to the terminal phalanx. This may be due to clubbing, finger nail clubbing, Heberden's nodes or terminal i.p. joint arthritis. What relevant physical signs are shown here? What is the diagnosis?

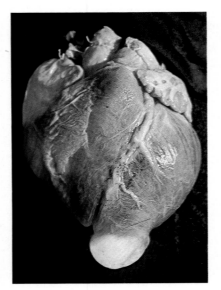

**48.** Post-mortem examination of a Brazilian revealed this apical aneurysm. What parasitic disease could produce this condition?

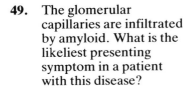

**49.** The glomerular capillaries are infiltrated by amyloid. What is the likeliest presenting symptom in a patient with this disease?

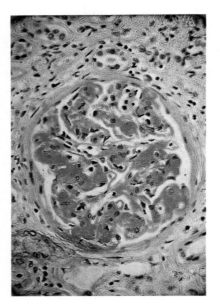

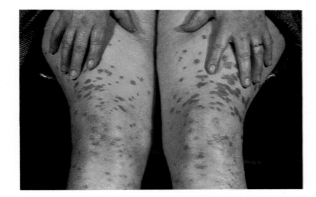

**50.** A patient with a skin rash developed a progressive arthritis involving the terminal phalanges particularly. The most likely diagnosis is which of the following?

a) Disseminated lupus erythematosis
b) Psoriasis
c) Lichen Planus
d) Diffuse sarcoidosis
e) E. Coli Septicaemia

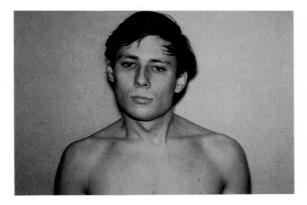

**51.** The young teenager cannot fully turn his head to the left. The left sternomastoid muscle is taut and inurated. What is the diagnosis?

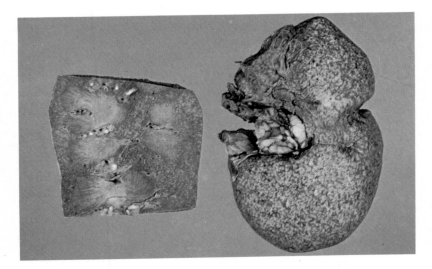

**52.** The combination of renal shrinkage, and severe atherosclerosis of intra-renal arteries is characteristic of which underlying disease?

**53.** This X-ray picture is typical of which of the following?

   a) A bilateral lung contusion
   b) A right heart hypertension
   c) Pulmonary fat embolism

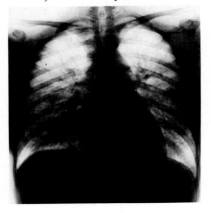

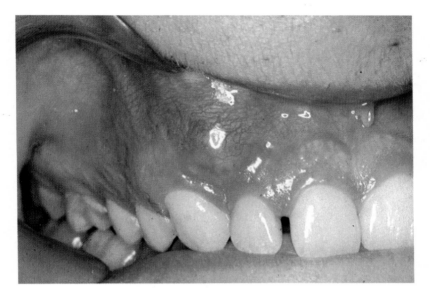

54. Expansion of the alveolar process with a bluish cast to the mucosa and displacement of adjacent teeth normally are signs associated with what?

55. While bathing this 3-year-old boy the mother accidentally discovered an abdominal mass. What is the most likely cause? What is the prognosis?

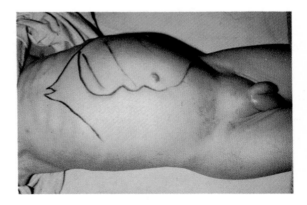

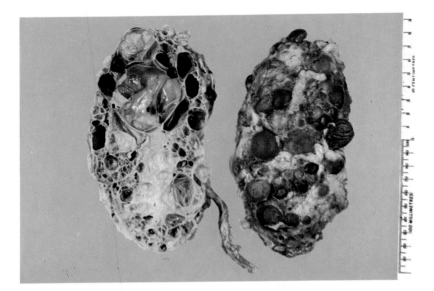

**56.** Which form of renal disease is illustrated in this hemisected specimen and what is a common presenting symptom of this disorder?

**57.** What is this condition?

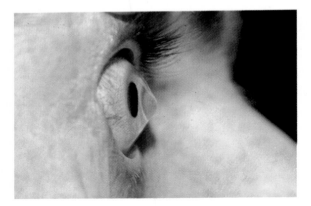

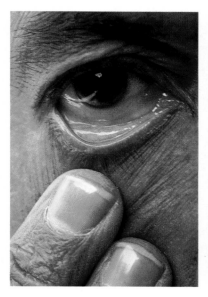 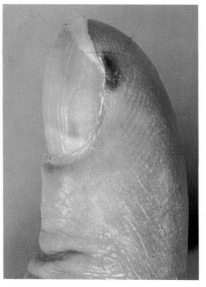

**58.** What is the significance of a polished nail? Here you notice jaundice of the sclera and a shiny nail tip. What are the causes of the shiny nail?

**59.** What is this lesion?

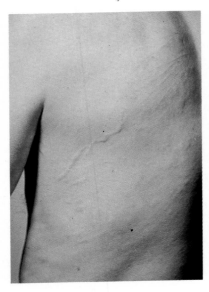 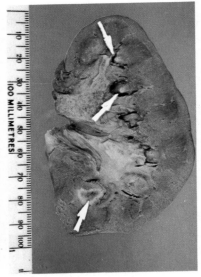

**60.** This soldier complained of recurrent, itching streaks on his trunk several years after he returned from jungle service in Malaysia. What is the diagnosis?

**61.** Arrows indicate lesions of renal papillae. Name the disease process involved and a clinical condition with which it is associated.

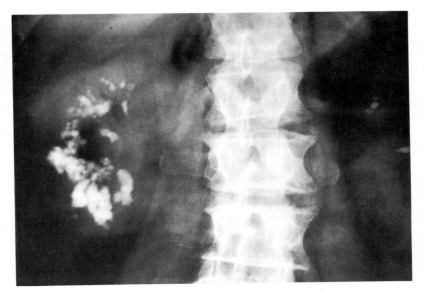

**62.** Radiographic evidence in this case draws attention to two co-existing diseases. Name them.

**63.** These are the genitalia of a mentally retarded male.

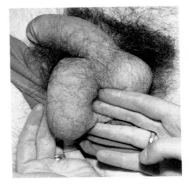

    a) What is the diagnosis?
    b) What tests would you ask for to confirm the diagnosis and what would you expect to find?

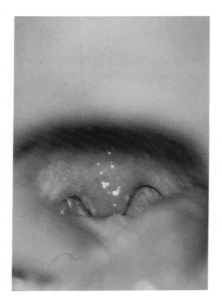

**64.** A teenager has a sore throat — his physician has noted pharyngitis and prescribed: What was the drug, the diagnosis and the error?

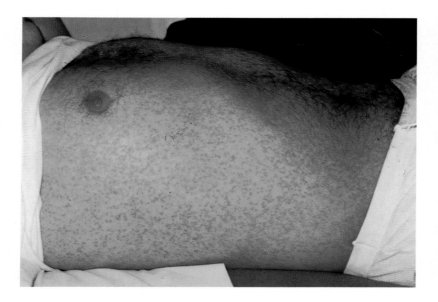

**65.** From what disease is this patient suffering?

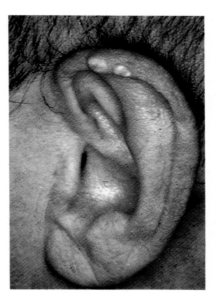

**66.** This girl started breast development (thelarche) at the age of two years without other pubertal changes. What is the prognosis?

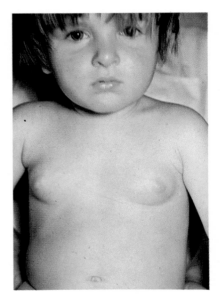

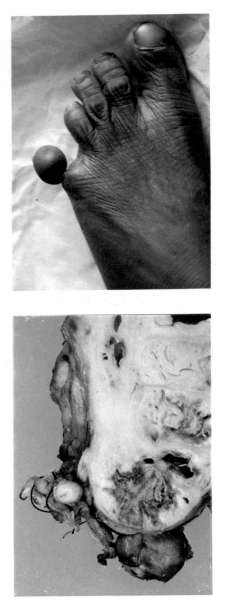

**67.** A curiosity — very common in Africa. What is it?

**68.** Gross appearances of this specimen may be confused with those of tuberculous renal disease. What is the disease in question?

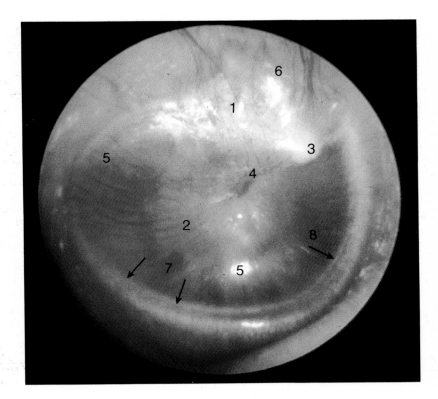

**69.** Name the numbered structures.

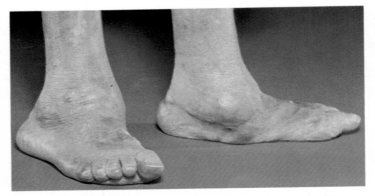

**70.** What disease are these foot deformities typical of?

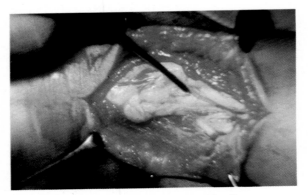

**71.** Of what is this an awful warning?

**72.** What clinical sign is shown here and what causes it?

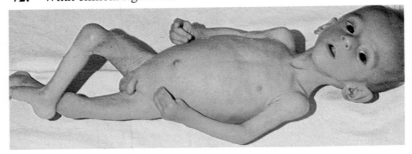

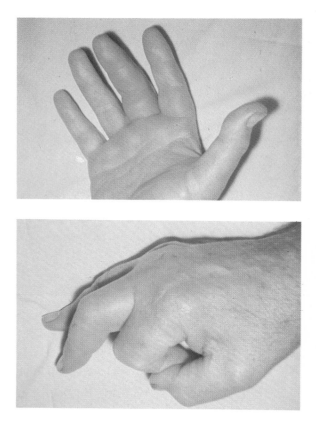

**73.** This veterinary surgeon presented five days after a cat had bitten him over the proximal interphalangeal flexion crease of his right middle finger. He had throbbing pain and swelling and stiffness. His right middle finger was swollen, red, warm, had a flexion deformity of the P.I.P. joint and there was tenderness over the flexor tendon sheath from the distal phalanx to the distal palm. Attempts to passively extend or flex the finger produced severe pain in the finger.

   a) What is the diagnosis?
   b) What is the treatment?

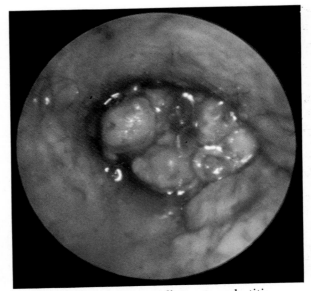

**74.** This patient was treated for a long-standing external otitis. After the infection had cleared, the otoscopic examination was as shown.

    a) What is your diagnosis?
    b) What would be your next step in making a diagnosis?

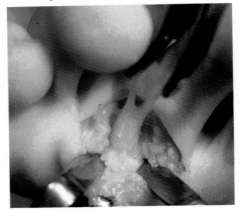

**75.** What is this? What are the symptoms?

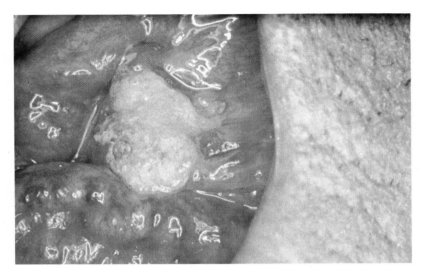

**76.** Papilliferous nodule on the floor of the mouth adjacent to the edentulous alveolus — what is the probable diagnosis?

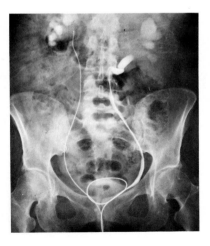

**77.** What is the condition associated with the following?

a) Bilateral hydronephrosis
b) Medical deviation of ureters
c) Ureteric catheters pass easily to renal pelves

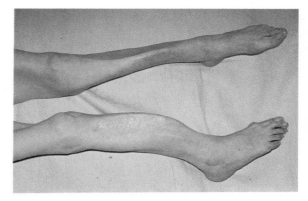

78. The deformity of the legs shown in the picture may occur in?

a) Chondrocalcinosis
b) Osteoporosis
c) Syphilis
d) Scurvy
e) Paget's disease

79. The lips (also finger tips and ears) may indicate the cause of intestinal obstruction — name the syndrome?

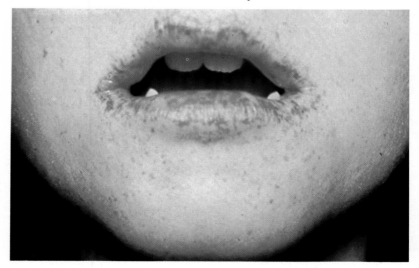

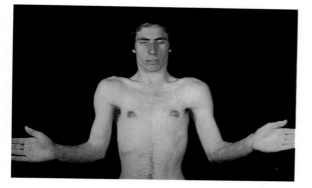

**80.** What does the discrepancy between powerful arms and loss of muscle bulk of the chest and the facial expression indicate?

**81.** The facial features of these babies are peculiar. Can you spot their condition?

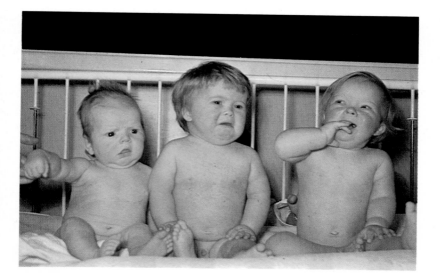

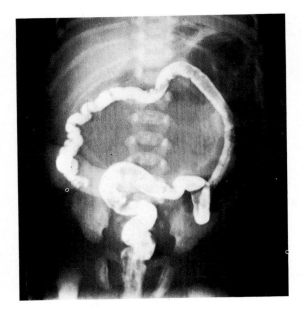

82. The enema on a patient with meconium peritonitis confirms which of the following statements about this condition?

a) May be asymptomatic
b) Is often found in the absence of overt perforation
c) May complicate cystic fibrosis
d) Can occur prenatally
e) Is seldom fatal

**83.** What is the nature of the lesion on the dorsum of this child's hand? What other clinical features should be sought in a child with this lesion?

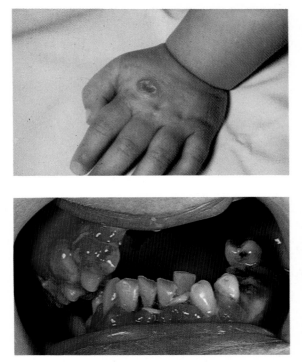

**84.** Changes in the gums of a 68-year-old woman patient with a fractured femur. The association could be due to which of the following?

a) Chronic sepsis
b) Epanutin dosage
c) Nifedipene dosage
d) Hyperparathyroidism
e) Hypoparathyroidism

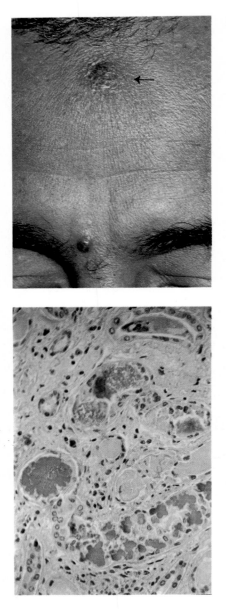

**85.** An area of pigmentation is present on this man's forehead. Is this occupational, malignant or cosmetic? A clue is that he was a religious man.

**86.** Laminated tubular casts, sometimes associated with giant cell reactions, granulomata and tubular disruption are found in cases of which systemic disorder?

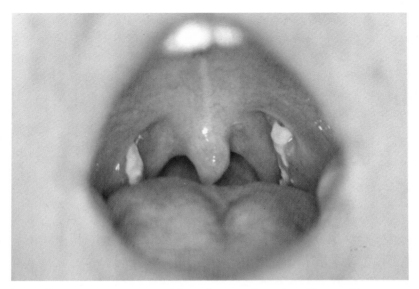

**87.** A young person complains of a sore throat and has not been immunised against diphtheria.

   a) Does he have diphtheria?

   b) What other physical signs would assist in differential diagnosis?

   c) What laboratory tests would confirm the diagnosis?

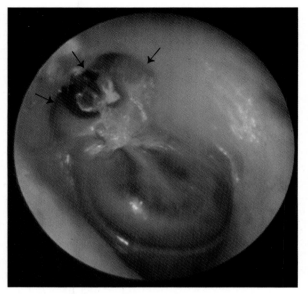

**88.** a) What is the diagnosis?
   b) What does the area labelled with the arrows designate?

**89.** Typical trophic ulcer at a pressure point, particularly prone to occur in diabetics. Why?

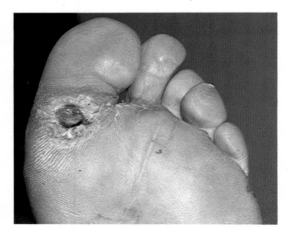

**90.** What is the cause of this facial swelling?

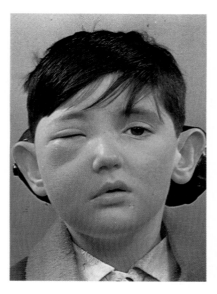

**91.** A coloured child is brought with a painful swollen finger. The winter has been cold. Could this be chilblains or is this trauma from a hammer, or has he been bitten by an insect? His brother also is jaundiced and anaemic. What blood investigations would you perform?

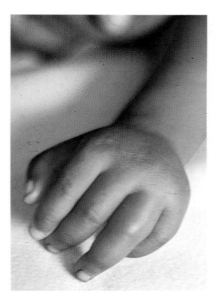

**92.** A holidaymaker develops a feverish illness on return from India. Apart from fever there is nothing to find on clinical examination except a few discrete pinkish macules on the abdomen.

a) Would the spots blanche on pressure?
b) Would they come out in crops?
c) Would the patient have a sore throat?
d) What is the most likely diagnosis?

**93.** This child complained of excruciating pain on defecation accompanied by rectal bleeding. What is the cause? How is the condition best managed and what are the consequences of inadequate treatment?

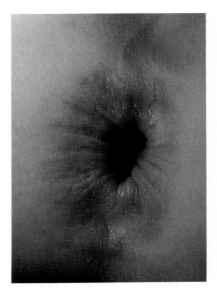

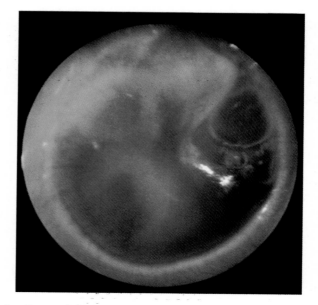

**94.**  a) What is the diagnosis?
   b) How much hearing loss would you expect in a patient with this condition?
   c) What are the likely causes of such a lesion?

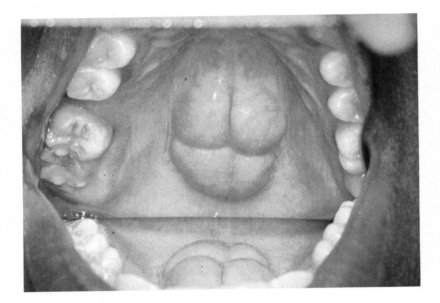

**95.** Bony hard fixed, lobulated, painless swelling in the midline forward of the back of the palate — What is the diagnosis?

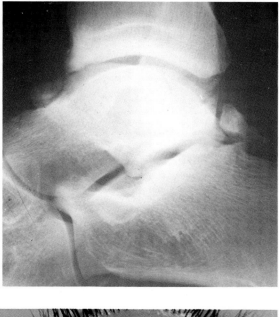

**96.** What is this?
What is it not?

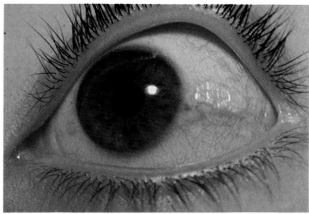

**97.** Whose name is associated with this lesion?
Is it pathognomonic of vitamin A deficiency?

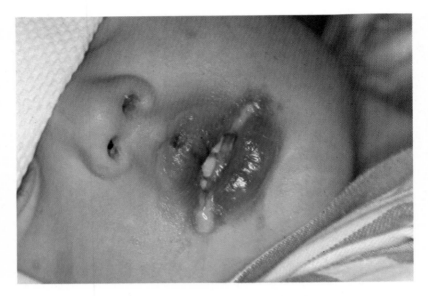

**98.** A young child becomes very unwell with a high fever and a painful mouth.

a) What is the likely diagnosis?
b) What is the causative organism?
c) What proportion of the child population possess antibody against the agent by the age of six years?

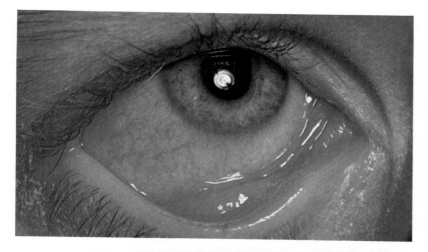

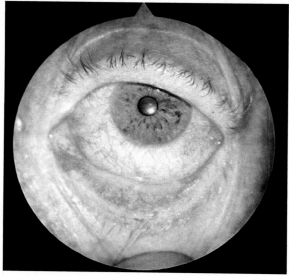

**99.** The patient complains of a sore, red eye of a few days duration. The other eye will be affected to a similar or lesser degree and the visual acuity is normal.

a) What is the diagnosis and how would you treat it?
b) In what circumstances would you refer it?

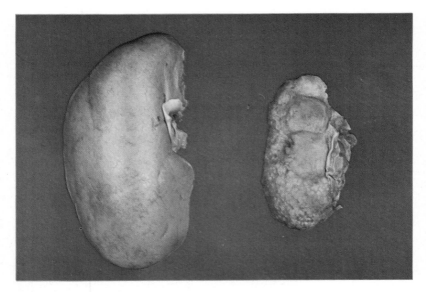

**100.** The normal kidney on the left contrasts with the scarred, contracted kidney on the right. The latter is characteristic of which disorder?

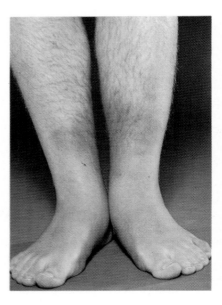

**101.** Tender red raised patches in the lower leg. What is the diagnosis?

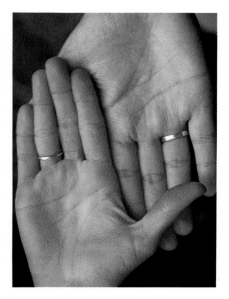

**102.** The right hand is a normal colour, the left hand is yellow, but the patient was not jaundiced. What is the differential diagnosis?

**103.** A woman develops a high fever and a painful skin eruption.

a) Would you expect her mucous membranes to be involved?
b) What is the diagnosis?
c) Name two possible causes.

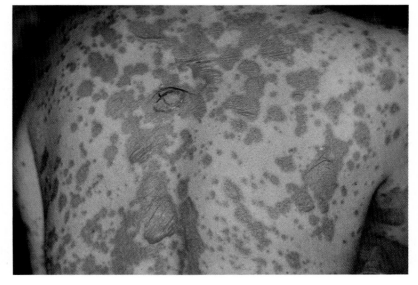

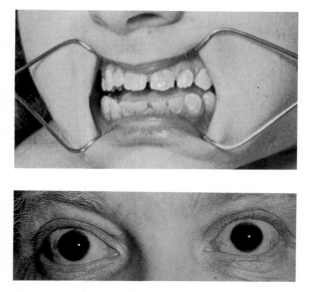

**104.** A 10-year-old boy shows imperfect dentition and markedly blue sclera. What is the probable diagnosis?

**105.** What was this injury and how was it treated?

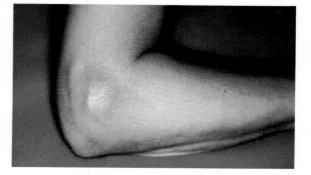

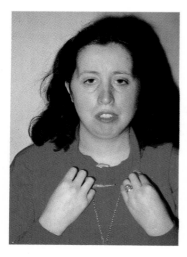

**106.**
a) Diagnosis in mother or child?
b) Recurrence risk for mother?
c) Mother's sister is worried about risks to her offspring — what tests would you do?
d) Is pre-natal diagnosis available?

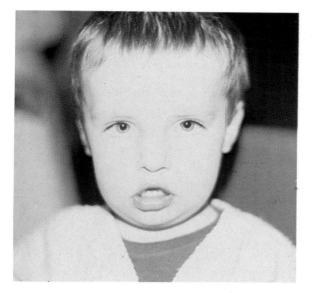

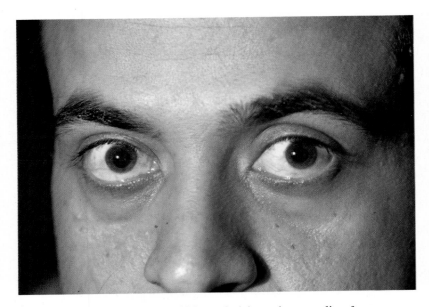

**107.** This man complains of blurred vision when reading from time to time, you examine him and notice that the right pupil does not contract on exposure to light. Why may this be? What other signs may be present? Why does he sometimes have difficulty in reading?

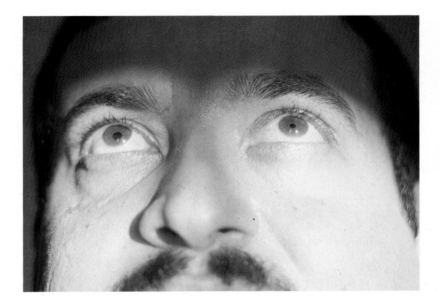

**108.** The lesion in the upper pole of this kidney is a typical example of which tumour?

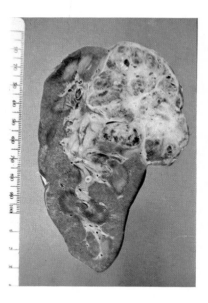

**109.** How may percutaneous biopsy benefit a patient with renal disease?

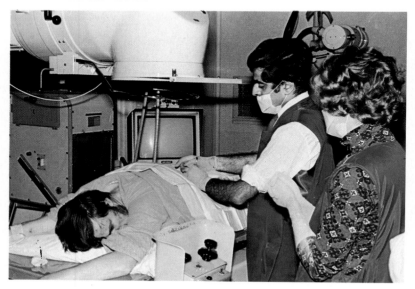

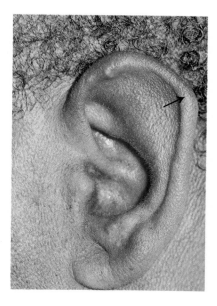

**110.** There are two prominences on the helix of this ear. The patient complains of intermittent severe pain in the left wrist. What are the two prominences due to? One might be metabolic, one might be atavistic.

**111.** The brain of this deceased indicates (or is compatible with) which of the following?

a) Parkinson's disease
b) Possible multiple sclerosis
c) Fat embolism

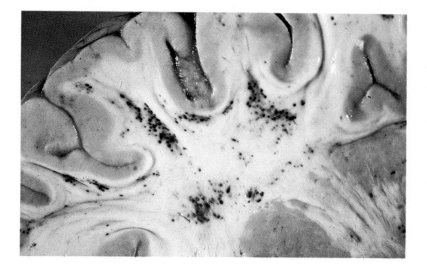

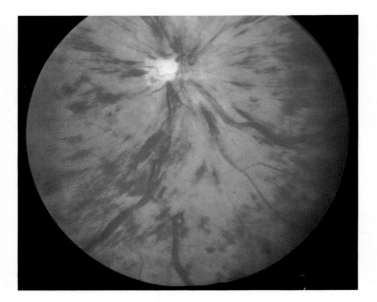

**112.**  a) List the retinal abnormalities shown in the illustration; what event do they signify?

  b) Which systemic disorders may be associated with this ocular condition?

**113.** Firm immobile, progressive painless swelling of the hard/ soft palate junction usually signifies what?

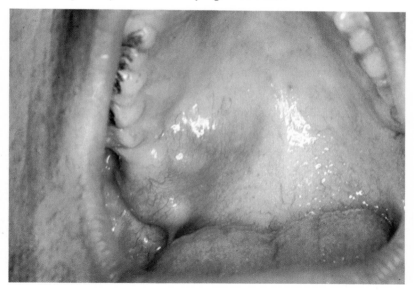

**114.** What is this sign?

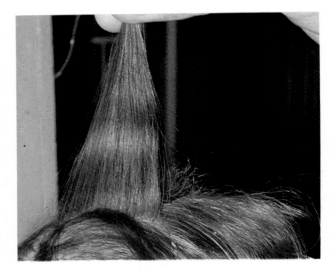

**115.** The mother of this male infant noted a swelling in the left groin when she was changing the child's napkin. What is the diagnosis and at what age should the infant be referred for treatment?

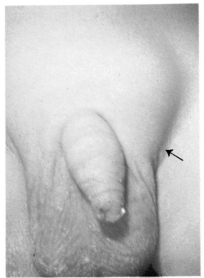

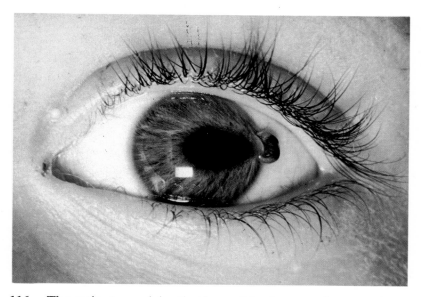

**116.** The patient complains that 'something has gone in my eye'.

    a) What further details do you wish to know in the history?
    b) What is the diagnosis and what would you do?

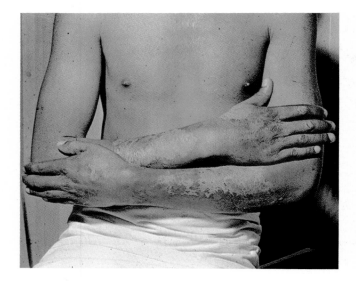

**117.** Bilaterally symmetrical photosensitive dermatosis is characteristic of what deficiency disease?

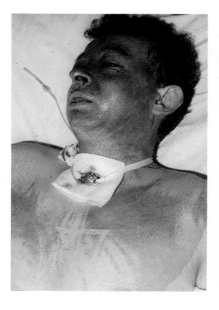

**118.** Such appearances are referred to as which of the following?

a) Mine-workman facies
b) Ecchymotic mask
c) Bywaters' crush-syndrome

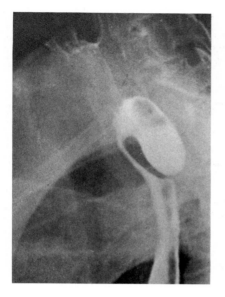

**119.** This pharyngeal pouch is commonly associated with which of the following?

a) An oesophageal neoplasm
b) Crico-pharyngeal webbing
c) Cervical osteo-arthritis
d) Hiatus Hernia

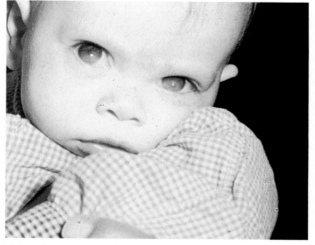

**120.** Bilateral central inferior corneal scars are suggestive of what prior deficiency?

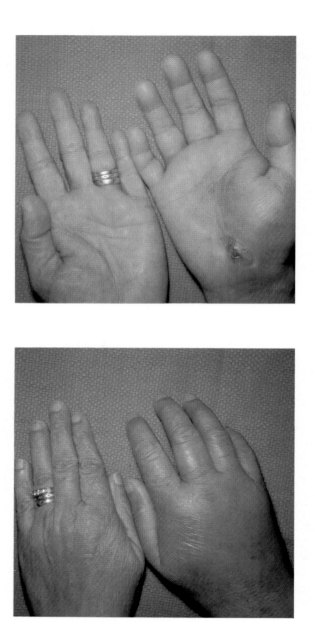

**121.** *History:* Four days after a puncture wound with a kitchen skewer this housewife presented with throbbing pain. *Examination:* Tenderness over the wound and the thenar eminence, slight discharge from the wound, swelling of the thenar eminence and dorsum of the hand and restricted thumb and index finger movement.

    a) What is the likely diagnosis?
    b) Is this cellulitis or suppuration?
    c) What is the treatment?

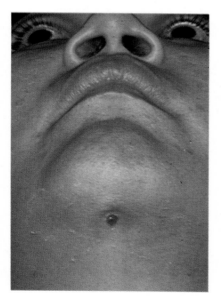

**122.** This persistent submental granulation is probably which of the following?

    a) Dental
    b) Tuberculosis
    c) An infected congenital sinus
    d) Secondary to a tongue lesion

**123.** The photograph shows a child with growth retardation and an age and sex-matched control.

a) What are the three commonest causes of short stature?

b) How can bone age estimation distinguish between short stature due to adrenocortical hyperactivity and growth hormone deficiency?

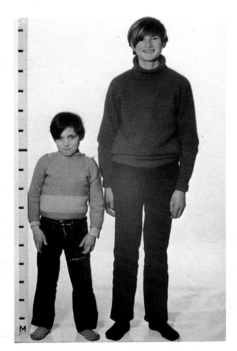

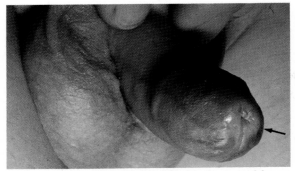

**124.** Following a number of episodes of balanitis this 8-year-old boy complained that he was unable to retract his foreskin. What is the diagnosis? What treatment should be recommended? Under what circumstances is this method of treatment contraindicated?

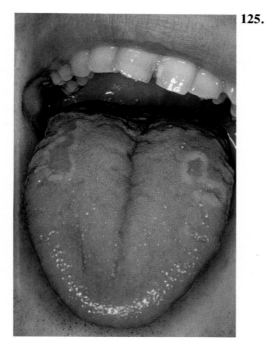

**125.** a) What is this common condition of the tongue?
b) Is it associated with generalised disease?
c) What is the treatment?

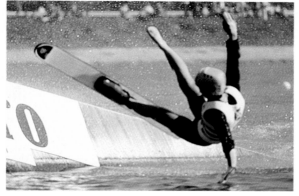

**126.** What peculiar risk does this sport hold for females?

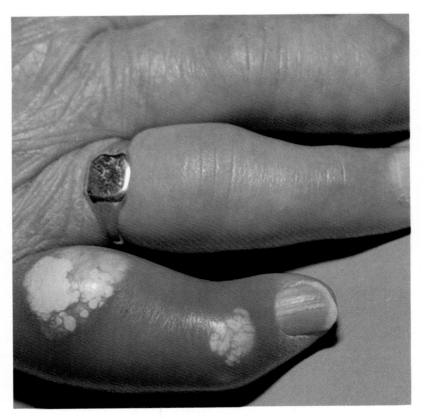

**127.** This 75-year-old female patient complained of pain in the fingers of right hand and fever. She has?

a) Bouchards nodes
b) Pseudo-gout
c) Rheumatoid nodule
d) Tophaceous gout
e) Hypertrophic pulmonary osteoarthropathy

**128.** This young girl developed a boil in the upper lip. This gradually increased in size and burst. The pus was evacuated by squeezing. She was admitted to hospital with high temperature, drowsiness and swelling of the eyelids. What complication is illustrated?

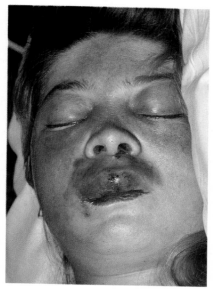

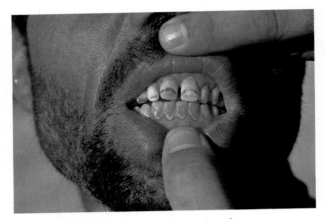

**129.** Bands of brown mottling of the teeth occur in what condition?

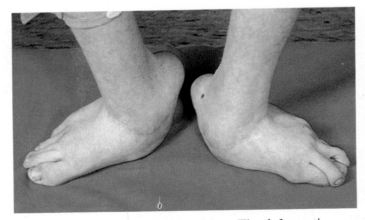

**130.** A young man with grossly deformed feet. The deformation cannot be passively corrected. What is he suffering from?

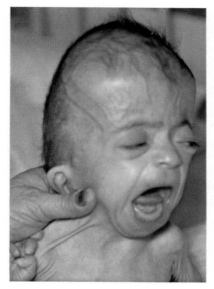

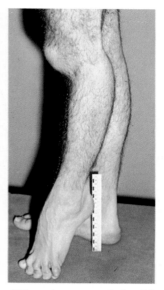

**131.** What is the name, pathology and prognosis of this cranial deformity?

**132.** A young adult with deformity of the left knee and gross shortening of the leg below the knee. What is the diagnosis?

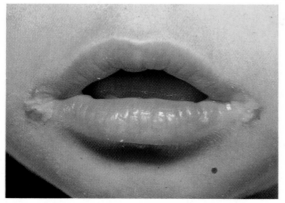

**133.** What are these angular lesions called?

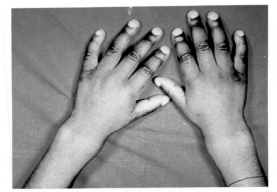

**134.** Swollen and painful wrists of a child. What is the diagnosis and how is it caused?

**135.** The condition shown is obviously a 'black eye' probably sustained by a blunt injury.
What other (a) ocular and (b) orbital injuries may also be present and how would you diagnose them?

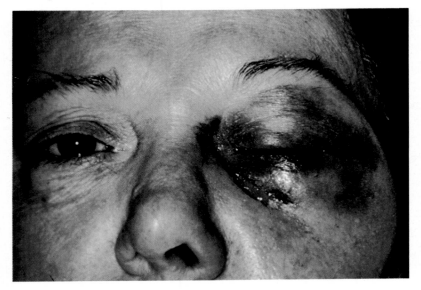

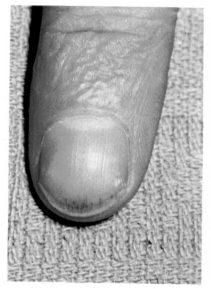

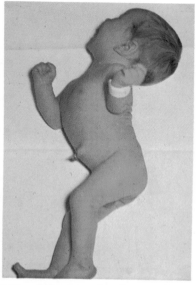

**136.** a) What is the term applied to these nail lesions?
   b) With what disease are they associated?

**137.** What are the diagnostic signs of this baby's condition?

**138.** Painful swelling in the perichondrium of the earlobe. What is the diagnosis?

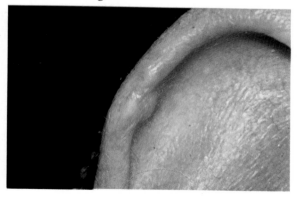

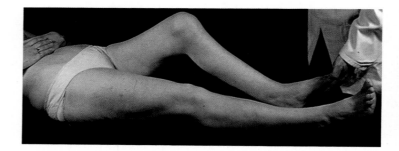

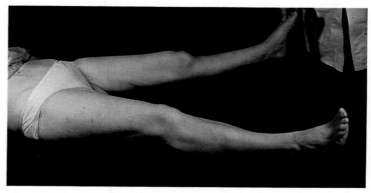

139. Flexion deformity of the left hip and left knee. Both deformities are corrected by simple abduction of left hip. How does this occur?

140. What is the diagnosis and what is the correct treatment for this condition?

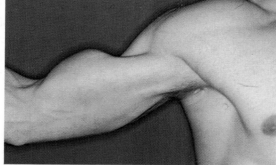

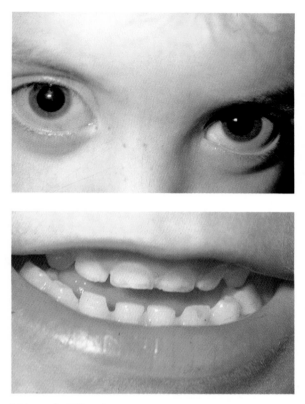

**141.** a) What features are shown here?
b) What is the diagnosis?

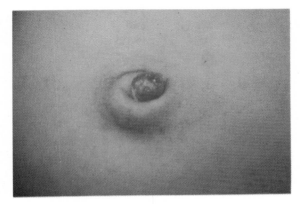

**142.** What is the diagnosis of the lesion in the umbilicus of a two-week-old baby? From what should it be differentiated? What is the treatment?

**143.** This hyperplastic gingivitis is drug induced.

  a) Of what treatment is it a well established complication?
  b) What other common state can lead to hyperplastic gingivitis?
  c) What is the treatment?

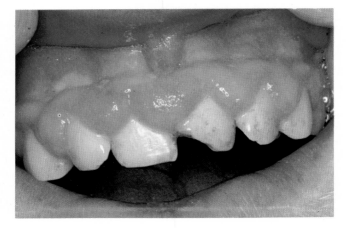

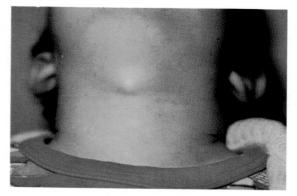

**144.** What is the diagnosis of this cystic swelling in the midline of the neck which moves on protruding the tongue? When should the child be referred for surgery?

**145.** This is a lesion of 6 months standing in an elderly male patient.

    a) What might it be?
    b) Is the clinical picture a typical one?
    c) With what is it often confused?

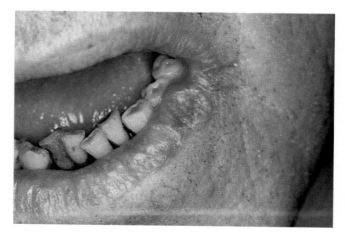

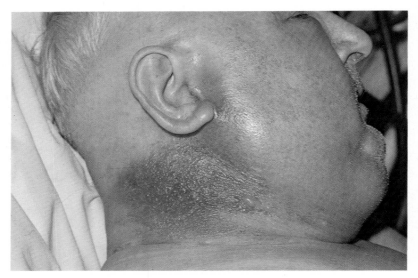

**146.** This man has an area of inflammation in his neck surrounded by severe oedema.

    a) Does he have erysipelas?
    b) Is it likely that an organism may be grown on blood culture?

**147.** Deformity of the left foot. What is it called, and how is it produced?

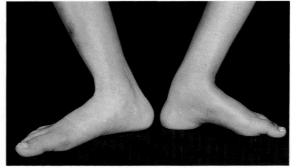

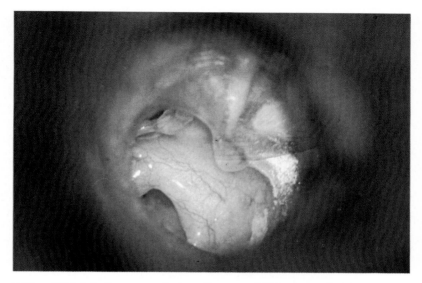

**148.** Which is the most obvious feature visible through this tympanic membrane perforation?

    a) Oval window    c) Incus
    b) Round window  d) Pyramid

**149.** a) Describe the abnormality shown
      b) Name the condition

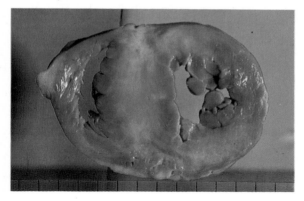

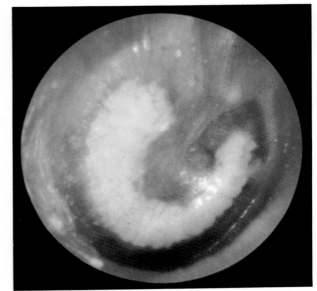

**150.** a) What is the diagnosis?
   b) What is the etiology of the chalky white plaques seen in the tympanic membrane?

**151.** The feet of a 25-year-old man showing deformity and pressure points under the heads of the metatarsal bones. What is this and how does it occur?

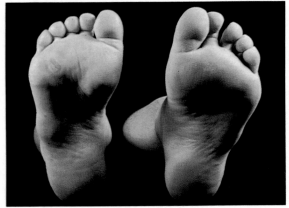

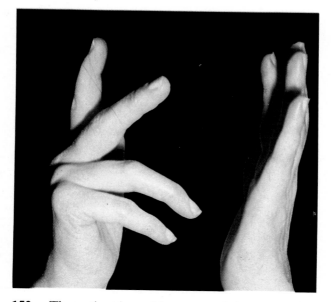

**152.** The patient is unable to extend the ring and little fingers of the right hand. What is this condition?

**153.** a) What can you deduce from this picture?
b) Can you suggest a reason for the patient being admitted to hospital?

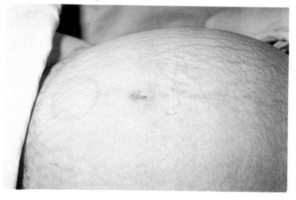

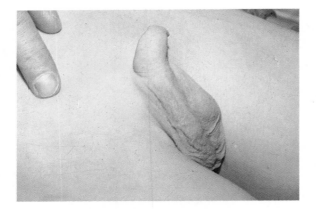

**154.** To what is the finger of the doctor referring? When is treatment best carried out? What are the dangers of delayed treatment? What are the possible long-term consequences?

**155.** *History:* Recurring pain and swelling over the radial portion of the left wrist, worse after movements of the thumb. *Examination:* Tender swelling over the radial portion of the wrist. Pain is aggravated by flexion of the thumb and simultaneous ulnar deviation of the wrist.

a) What is the differential diagnosis?
b) What is the treatment?

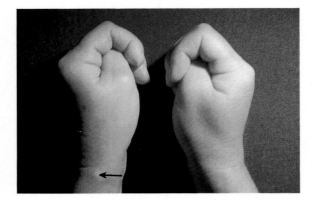

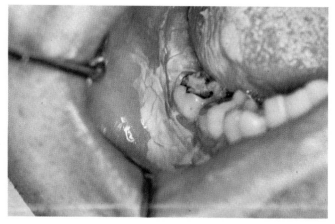

**156.** This patient complained of severe pain and the rapid appearance of this white patch.

    a) What might the origin of the patch be?
    b) What might be the origin of the pain?
    c) What is the treatment?

**157.** These overgrown toenails are a sign of?

    a) Alzheimer's disease
    b) Hallux valgus
    c) Psoriasis
    d) Neglect
    e) Peripheral vascular disease

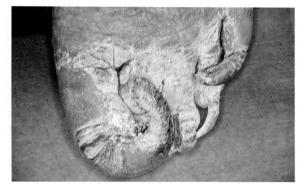

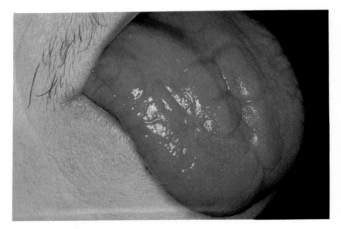

**158.** This is a patient with a haematological deficiency.

a) What might this be?
b) Is this a specific picture?
c) Would this occur early or late in the disease process?

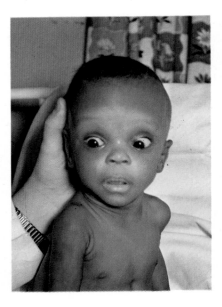

**159.** A five-year-old child; what does the look indicate?

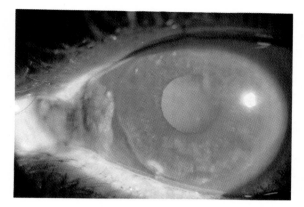

**160.** The fluorescein shows mucous tags on the cornea. What is the cause?

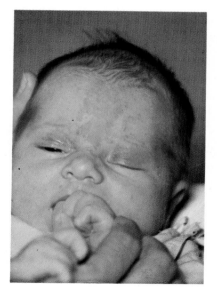

**161.** Newborn with unilateral naevus flammeus along the first branch of the trigeminus. What will the X-ray investigation of the skull disclose?

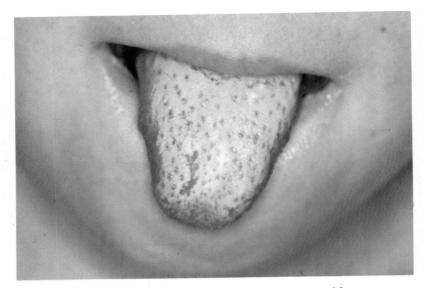

162. a) From the appearance of the tongue what would you consider to be the most likely diagnosis?
    b) What changes would you expect during the following few days?

163. a) What are the possible obstetrical and gynaecological diagnoses for the swelling?
    b) What simple test would you do to exclude a physiological cause?

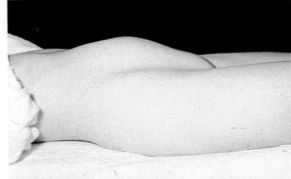

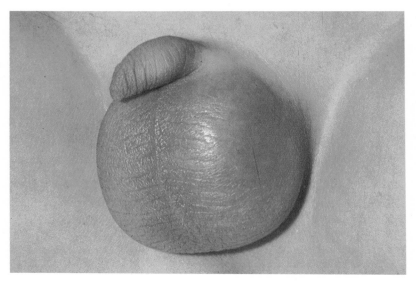

**164.** This young child of 7 years complained of lower abdominal pain of rapid onset. On examination the marked swelling and redness was obvious in the left side of the scrotum. What treatment should be instituted?

**165.** The patient presents with aching in the right buttock, general malaise and weight loss. The swelling in the buttock is fluctuant. What is the diagnosis?

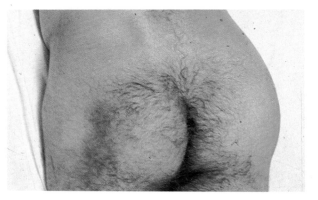

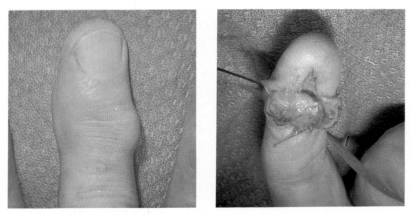

**166.** *History:* Gradual increase in swelling at the distal inter-phalangeal joint.
*Examination:* A firm subcutaneous swelling in the area of the distal inter-phalangeal joint.

  a) What is the differential diagnosis?
  b) What investigations?
  c) What is the treatment?

**167.** The shoulder is obviously grossly wasted and disorganised. There are abnormal neurological signs in the left upper limb. What is the diagnosis?

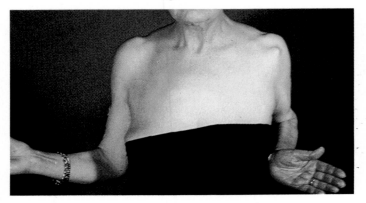

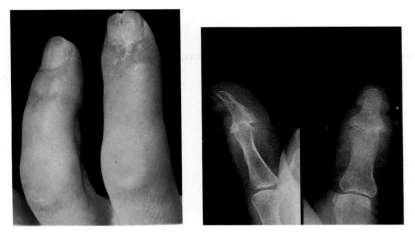

**168.** A chronic low grade inflammatory reaction of the nailbed with splitting of the nail. There are few scattered skin lesions elsewhere in the body. X-ray shows destruction of the distal inter-phalangeal joints. What is the diagnosis?

**169.** The patient complained of vaginal discharge and irritation. What is the cause with the cervix and posterior fornix exposed? Why does the discharge usually contain small bubbles? What treatment would you suggest?

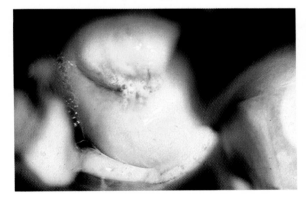

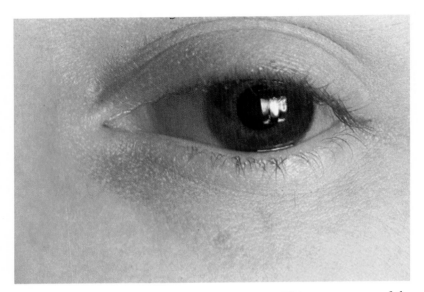

**170.** This appearance of the eye may be associated with hereditary dental abnormalities; to what may the patient be especially predisposed?

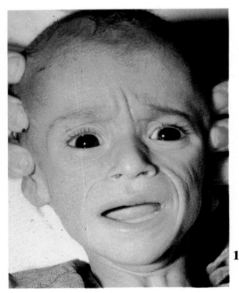

**171.** What is this appearance called and what causes it?

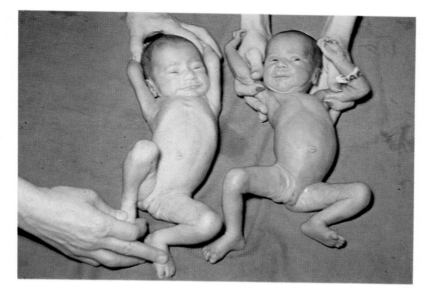

**172.** Monozygous monochorionic twins. What caused the difference of their colour and development?

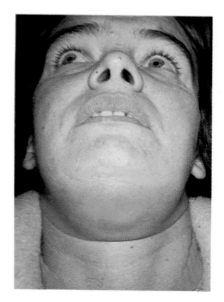

**173.** This tender midline neck swelling is suggestive of which of the following?

  a) An infected thyro-glossal cyst
  b) Ludvig's angina
  c) A plunging ranula
  d) A furuncle

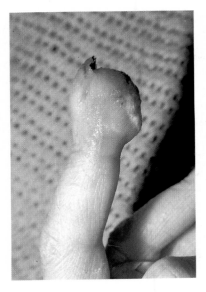

**174.** *History:* This 60-year-old man presented with a six month history of an inflamed swollen fingertip.
*Examination:* There was a fungating tumour at the fingertip.

  a) What is the differential diagnosis?
  b) Investigations?
  c) What treatment?

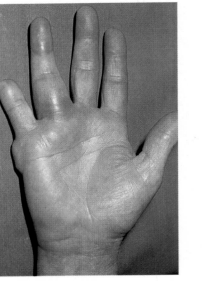

**175.** *History:* Recurring pain, swelling and redness of the right ring finger. No history of injury.
*Examination:* Redness, swelling and increased warmth. Restricted movement.

  a) What is the differential diagnosis?
  b) What investigations?
  c) What treatment?

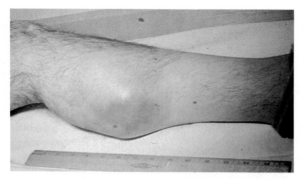

**176.** A young man with painful enlarged swelling of the right calf. There is a history of excessive bleeding following dental extraction. What is the diagnosis?

**177.** This swelling of the lower lip may be associated with gastrointestinal disease.

   a) What might this be?
   b) What other oral lesions may occur?
   c) What is the management of these patients?

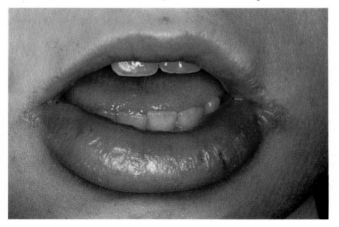

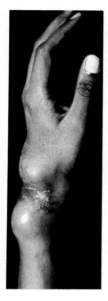

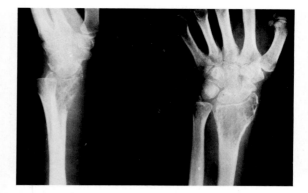

**178.** A 'dumbbell' tumour straddling under the extensor retinaculum of the wrist of an 18-year-old boy. Radiographs show a destructive lesion of the lower end of the radius. What is the diagnosis?

**179.** This female patient complained of painful feet and recurrent falls. Examination of the foot shows?

a) Bunion
b) Hallux Valgus
c) Nail dystrophy
d) Koilonychia
e) Hammer toes

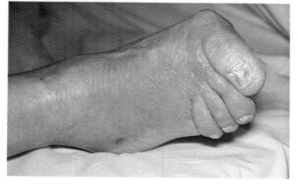

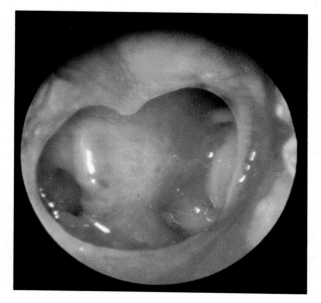

**180.** a) What is the diagnosis?
    b) What organisms would you expect if this ear were cultured?
    c) Would you choose systemic or topical antibiotics for this infection?

**181.** What is the cause of these subcutaneous depressions?

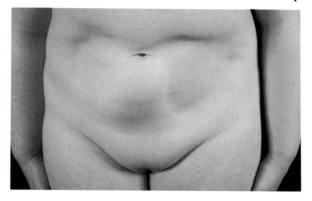

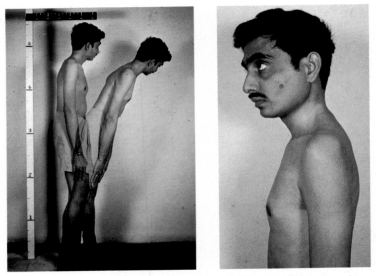

**182.** The young man is trying to touch his toes. His spine does not bend at all and he can barely reach his toes with his fingertips. On attempting to turn his head the patient turns his eyes outwards but the neck is held rigidly. What is the diagnosis?

**183.** Indolent, painless lesions occurring on the shins of young person. What is the underlying disorder?

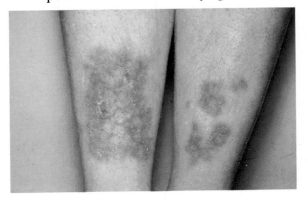

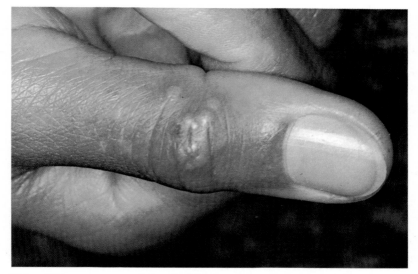

**184.** This nurse complained of feeling unwell with feverishness and headache. On examination she had a painful cluster of small blisters on her thumb.

    a)  What is the cause of the blisters?

    b)  Is the condition an occupational risk?

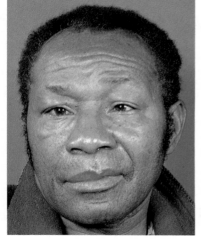

**185.** Double vision on looking to the right. Why?

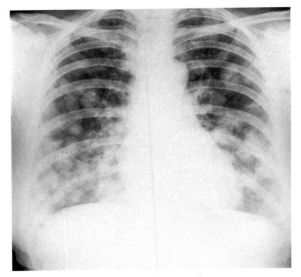

**186.** a) Describe the abnormality.
   b) Discuss the differential diagnosis.
   c) How do you establish the diagnosis?
   d) What is the treatment?

**187.** Large, oedematous, plethoric baby delivered at 38 weeks. What was at fault?

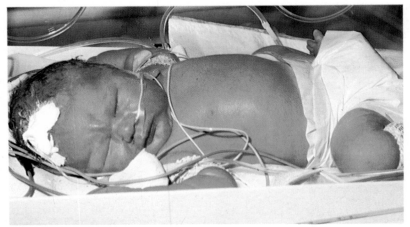

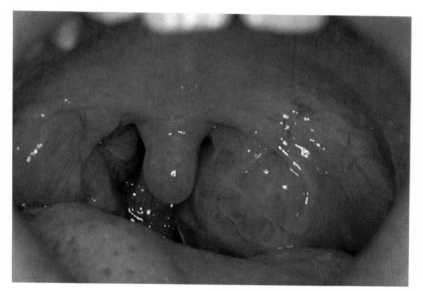

**188.** This large painless tonsil is indicative of which of the
following?
    a) Suggestive of infection
    b) Related to a parapharyngeal mass
    c) Suspicious of a tonsillar neoplasm
    d) Related to a tension cyst

**189.** a) An unusual
chest X-ray
appearance.
Describe what
you see.
    b) Explain the
appearance.
    c) Describe the
complications.

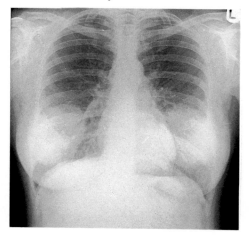

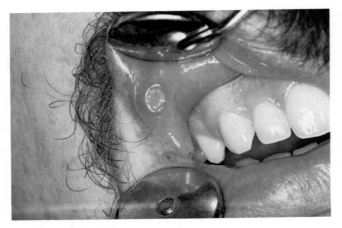

**190.** This is a common condition.

    a) What is the most likely diagnosis?
    b) What important differential diagnosis must be considered?
    c) What abnormality of the gastrointestinal tract maybe associated with it?

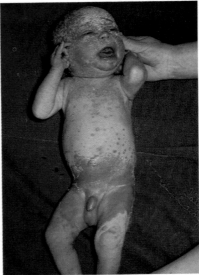

**191.** Name the baby's skin condition and prognosis.

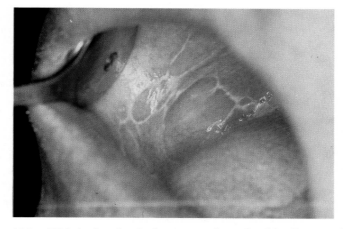

**192.** This is the classical presentation of a skin disease affecting the mouth.

    a) What is this?
    b) What other variants of the oral lesions may occur?
    c) What is the principle of treatment?

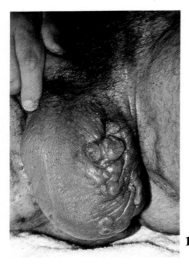

**193.**    Scrotal lesion. What is its causation?

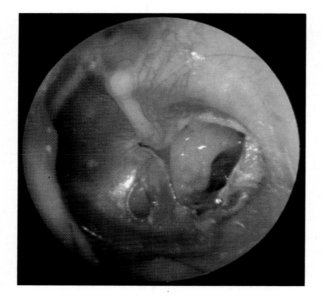

**194.** a) This left tympanic membrane was perforated by a blow to the side of the head. What is the dark structure seen through the larger of the two perforations?

b) What is the treatment of this type of perforation?

**195.** What abnormalities are shown in this eye of an elderly man?

a) Ectropion
b) Gerontoxon
c) Kayser-Fleischer ring
d) Exophthalmos
e) Holmes-Adie pupil

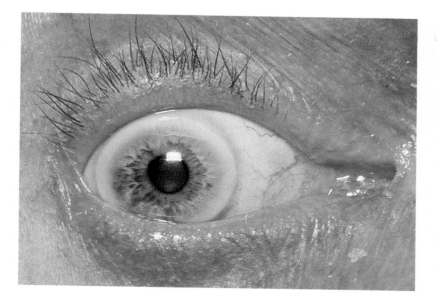

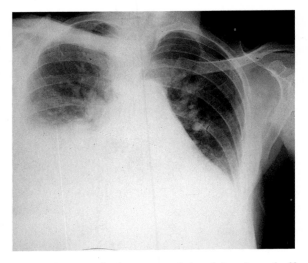

**196.**  a) What is the cause of the right pleural effusion?
b) As a rule, the diagnosis is confirmed by aspiration of fluid and pleural biopsy. Is it necessary in this instance?
c) If not, why not?
d) How is the diagnosis established?
e) Who is the disorder named after?
f) What are the complications?
g) What is the treatment?

**197.** *History:* Recurrent discharge of clear viscid fluid from beneath the nail fold of the middle finger. Recurring swelling over the extensor aspect of the D.I.P. joint. *Examination:* Horizontal ridging of the nail. A tender translucent swelling over the distal inter-phalangeal joint.

a) What is the diagnosis?
b) What is the treatment?

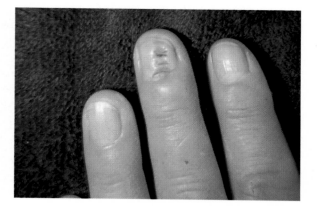

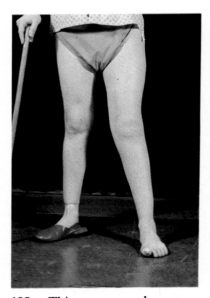

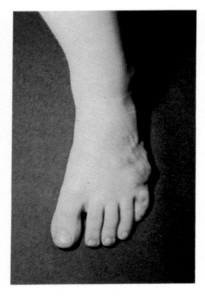

**198.** This young man has an elongated enlarged left lower limb with a soft bluish vascular tumour on the outer aspect of the foot. What is the diagnosis?

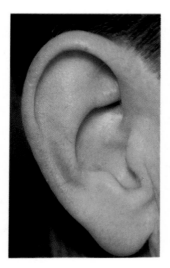

**199.** Earlobe showing bluish transparency of the cartilage. What is the disorder?

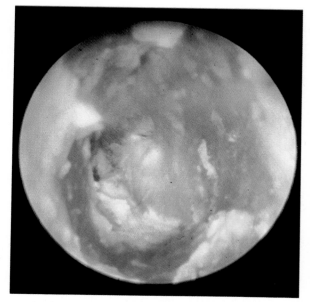

**200.** a) This otoscopic view represents which condition?

b) The most common bacterial causes of this condition are?

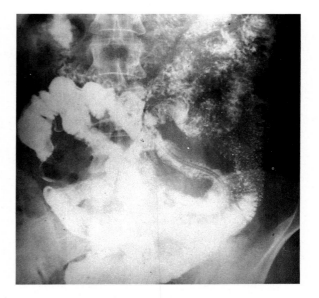

**201.** a) This patient has vague longstanding abdominal pain.
This is one of many barium meal examinations
performed on her. Describe the appearances?
b) What is the diagnosis?
c) How do you confirm the diagnosis?
d) What is the treatment?

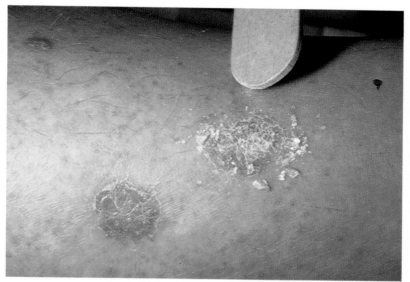

**202.** Red and scaly lesions are commonly seen in which of the following?

   a) psoriasis
   b) pityriasis rosea
   c) secondary syphilis
   d) urticaria
   e) ringworm infection

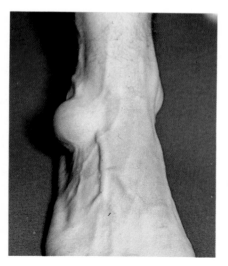

**203.** Painless globular swelling on the outer side of the ankle which was fluctuant on palpation. What is the diagnosis?

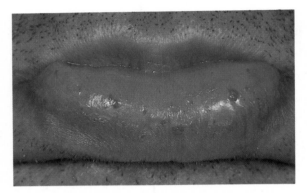

204. Which of the following might be associated with this patient's skin condition?

a) A positive serum antinuclear factor
b) Glycosuria
c) Raised serum immunoglobulin M
d) Scabies infection
e) Chronic renal failure

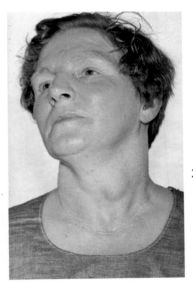

205. a) What is the diagnosis?
b) Which tests are likely to be most valuable in determining management?

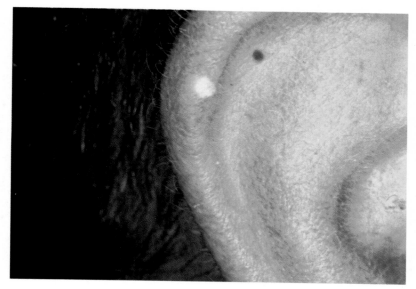

**206.** This aural lesion requires:

a) Excision/biopsy
b) Antibiotic/cortico-steroid ointment
c) Serology
d) Further investigation

**207.** Young woman with deteriorating vision. What is the cause?

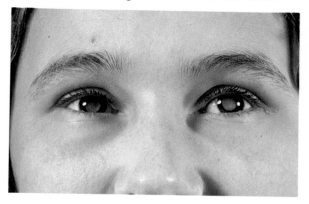

6 Plerlph Ploper What
A B C F H J I K                                    11/7/78

        ☆ 6 ~~Traaaph~~ Prmley Prakas
A B C D H I J K M N O T                             18/7/78.

        did
What this came from
What this it~~g~~~~ ~~ treatment

~~Th~~ir till
will ~~~~ come back                                23/7/78
will ~~~~ ~~~~ ~~~~
I b find a diff~~~~cult to spell

**208.**  a) What is this condition called and how is it defined?
          b) What is its anatomical significance?
          c) What are the most common causes?

**209.** Which of the following tests would be useful in confirming the cause of this girl's jaundice?

a) Serum hepatitis B surfacen antibody
b) Serum hepatitis B core antibody
c) Serum hepatitis A IgM antibody
d) Reticulocyte count
e) Test for urinary urobilinogen

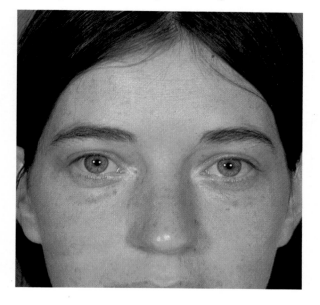

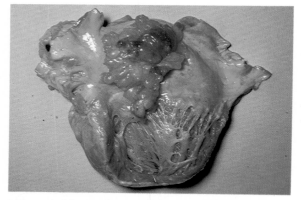

**210.**  a) Name the condition present in the left ventricle?
    b) Name its commonest site of origin?
    c) Describe the histological appearance of the condition?

**211.**  A nine months history of chronic fungus infection of the thumb around the nail.

  a) What is the differential diagnosis?
  b) What is the treatment?

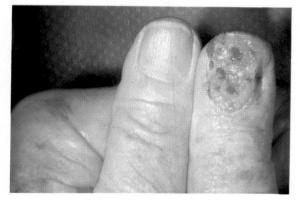

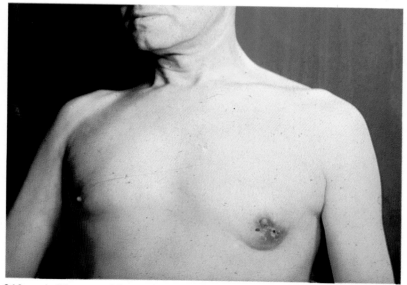

**212.** A 55-year-old man noted a small area of thickening below the left nipple. It gradually increased in size and in four months it was reddened yet painless, and the skin broke down over it. He was referred for surgery. What is the likely diagnosis?

**213.** a) Name the condition affecting the valve?
b) Describe the appearance of the valve?

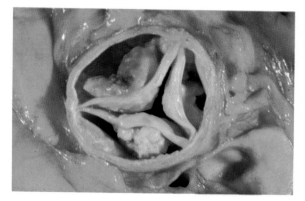

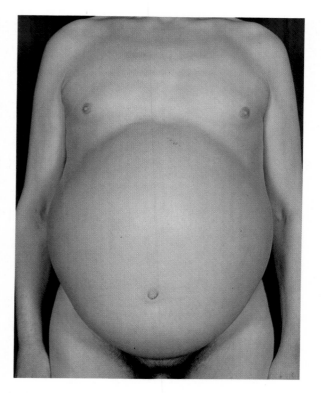

**214.** Which of the following might be useful in this patient?

a) Dietary sodium supplements
b) Chest X-ray
c) Dietary potassium supplements
d) Diagnostic abdominal paracentesis
e) Daily weight chart

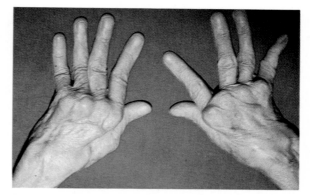

**215.** All the joints of this old lady's hands are disorganised. The metacarpophalangeal joints are the main site of disease. What is this disease?

**216.** This nasal vestibulitis is related to:

    a) Eczema elsewhere
    b) Maxillary sinusitis
    c) A self-induced lesion ('picking')
    d) A foreign body

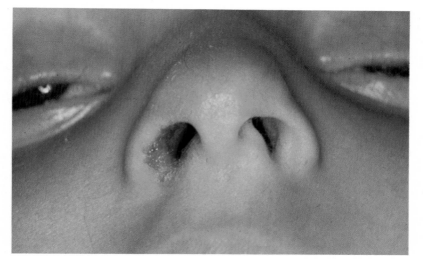

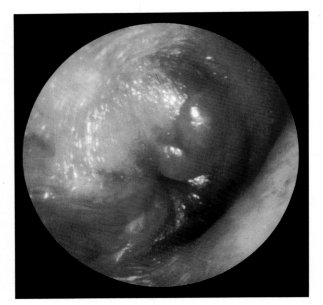

**217.** a) What is this extremely painful condition of the tympanic membrane called?

b) What is the etiology of this condition thought to be?

**218.** What is this condition of the cornea?

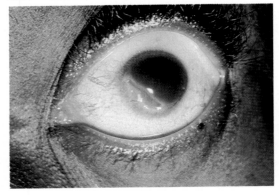

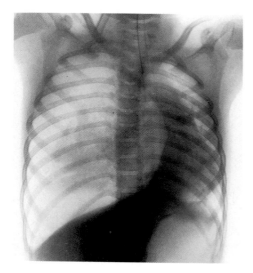

**219.** Which of the following is featured?

  a) A left haemothorax
  b) A right tension pneumothorax
  c) A pericardial tamponade

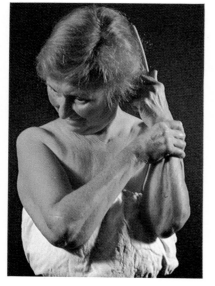

**220.** The patient is unable to comb her hair with her left hand without supporting it with the right hand. She has severe pain. From what is she suffering?

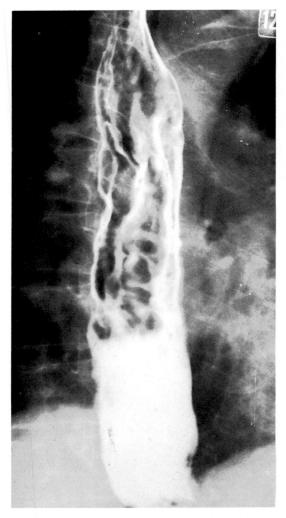

**221.** Which of the following might be in the patient who had this barium swallow radiography?

a) Monihasis of the mouth
b) Splenomegaly
c) Leukocytosis
d) Macrocytosis
e) Hepatic encephalopathy

**222.** Dermatological lesions often presenting as rings are which of the following?

a) granuloma annulare
b) erythema annulare centrifugum
c) pityriasis rosea
d) lichen planus
e) tinea corporis

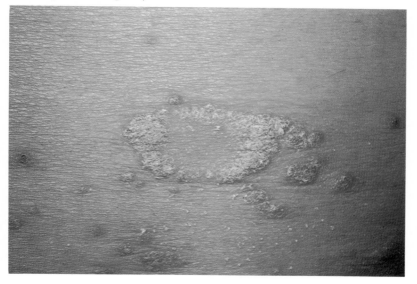

**223.** This narrowing of the external auditory meatus is due to:

a) Congenital atresia
b) Past fracture of the ear canal
c) Swimming
d) Stenous following otitis externa

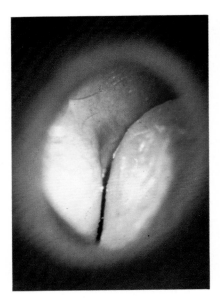

**224.** The diagnosis of these persistent raised very itchy patches on the nape is:

a) a fungal infection
b) allergic contact dermatitis
c) lichen planus
d) lichen simplex
e) scabies

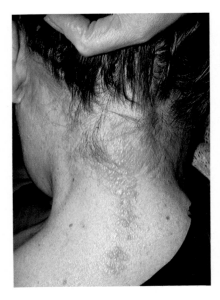

**225.** The boy in the picture has a progressive movement disorder (dystonia):

   a) What is the diagnosis?
   b) How will you confirm this?
   c) Can it be detected prenatally?

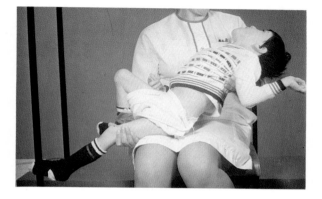

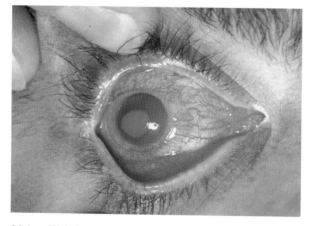

**226.** This is a severe ammonia burn of the eye a few days after a criminal assault. What is the prognosis?

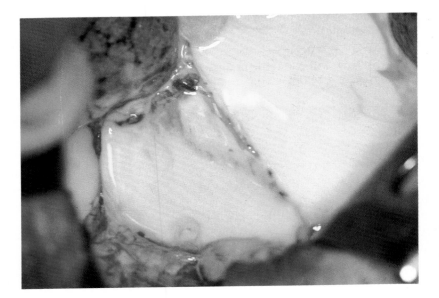

**227.** Which of the following is most likely?

    a) Typical staphylococcic pus from an empyema
    b) A chylothorax when opening the pleural cavity
    c) Peritonitis due to colic perforation

**228.** What is the abnormality and why?

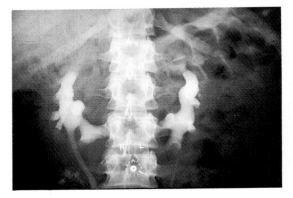

**229.** The organism which causes a 'stye' (hordeolum) is which of the following?

    a) staphylococcus epidermidis
    b) staphylococcus aureus
    c) streptococcus pyogenes
    d) herpes simplex
    e) corynebacterium acnes

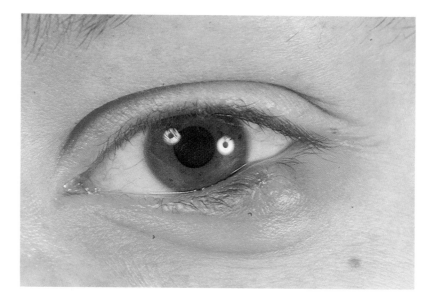

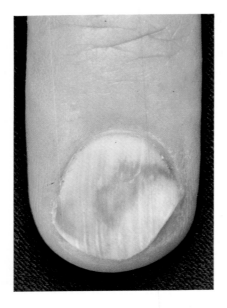

**230.** This nail plate shows nail separation (onycholysis) and redness typical of which of the following?

a) ringworm infection
b) candida infection
c) acute paronychia
d) a subungual tumour
e) psoriasis

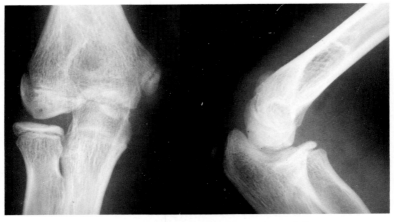

**231.** What is wrong here and what is the prognosis?

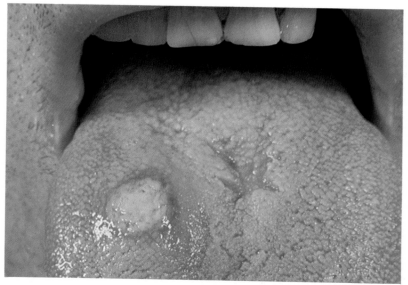

**232.** This superficial tender tongue ulcer is probably which of the following?

a) Luetic      c) A fungal lesion
b) Traumatic   d) Aphthous

**233.** What is the cause of this type of palpebral conjunctivitis?

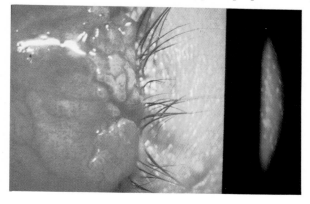

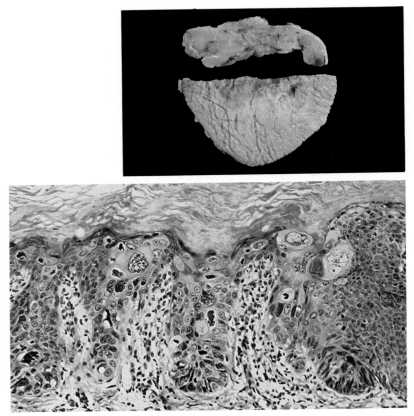

**234.** This scaly, slightly raised plaque on the inner aspect of the right leg of a 75-year-old woman has been present for several years, slowly enlarging. The section shows disorderly arrangement of epithelial cells with bizarre giant nuclei and with abnormal mitoses. The subjacent stroma shows scattered round cell infiltrate. Indicate which of the following is the correct clinical diagnosis.

a) Extramammary Paget's Disease  d) Borst Jadassohn's Disease
b) Bowen's Disease  e) Mycosis fungoides
c) Melanocarcinoma in situ  f) Junctional naevus

    Why would a pathologist examine many sections from such a lesion before issuing his report?

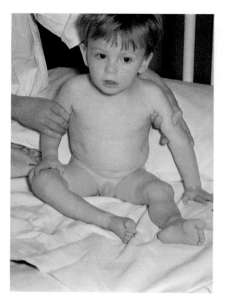

**235.** A two-year-old boy with freckles and patches of eczema has had tremor and convulsions since the age of six months. An elder sister is mentally retarded. What substance will be found in the urine?

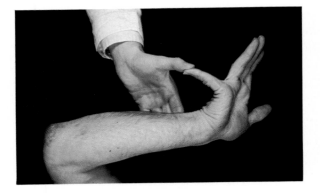

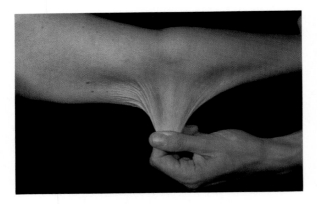

**236.** All the joints are excessively mobile and the skin is very lax. What is the diagnosis?

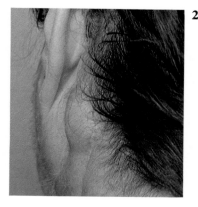

237. A woman patient with chronic renal failure had lumps appear behind her ears which were painless, but her joints became stiffer. The patient could be suffering from which of the following?

a) An infected scalp
b) Carcinomatosis
c) Tumoural calcinosis
d) Rheumatoid arthritis
e) Tuberculosis

238. Sudden exacerbation of gravitational dermatitis can result from which of the following?

a) viral infection
b) fungal infection
c) bacterial infection
d) a drug reaction
e) allergic contact sensitization

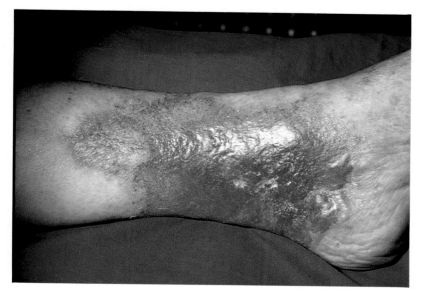

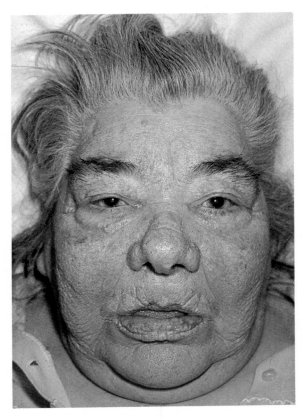

**239.** Which of the following clinical features would you expect to find in this case?

    a) Increased sensitivity to cold
    b) Ataxia
    c) Foot drop
    d) Hoarseness of voice
    e) Depression

**240.** *History:* This patient sustained a 3mm cut over the P.I.P. flexion crease of his left middle finger. There was spurting of blood from the wound.
*Examination:* A tidy wound with inability to actively flex the P.I.P. or D.I.P. joints. Numbness over the radial portion of the pulp.

a) What is the diagnosis? What deep structures may have been divided?
b) What is the treatment?

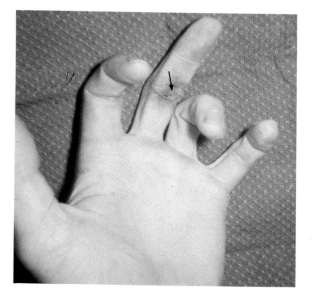

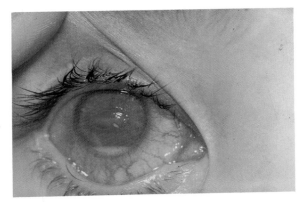

**241.** What is the diagnosis?

**242.** a) What is this syndrome?
b) What are the clinical features?
c) The parents are normal. What is the risk of further affected children?

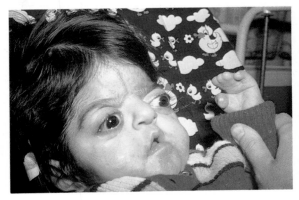

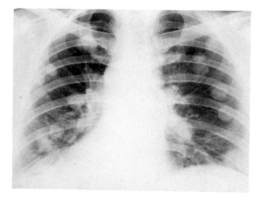

**243.** CXR showing what?

**244.** Pitted lesions of the nail plates may be seen in which of the following?

a) eczema  
b) psoriasis  
c) lichen polanus  

d) alopecia areata  
e) ringworm of nails  

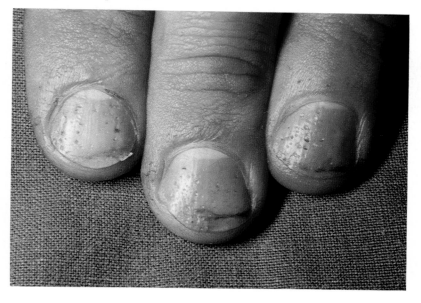

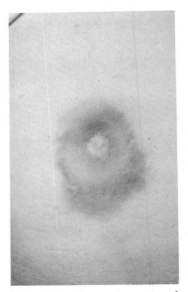

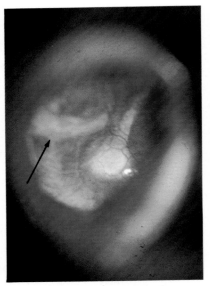

**245.** Discolouration around the umbilicus. Whose name was given to this sign? What is the underlying cause of the discolouration?

**246.** Which of the following does this white line visible on the tympanic membrane represent?

    a) A fluid level
    b) Cholesteatoma
    c) The chorda tympani
    d) The incus

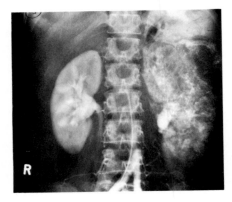

**247.** Haematuria, pain in the left loin, presence of mass. What does this arteriogram show?

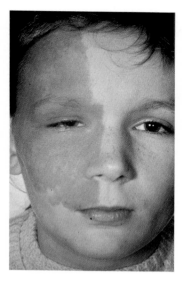

**248.**
a) What is the diagnosis?
b) What is the recurrence risk for her offspring?
c) She has Jacksonian epilepsy — on which side?
d) Describe how her skull X-ray might look?
e) Name one important ophthalmological complication?

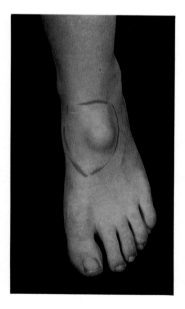

**249.** This patient has a painless swelling on the dorsum of his left foot. It is soft and semi-fluctuant. He has similar swellings elsewhere on his body, and there are patches of pigmentation of the skin. What is the diagnosis?

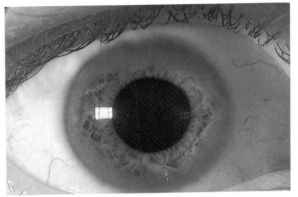

**250.** With which of the following might these appearances in the eye be associated?

a) Choreoathetosis
b) Hyperuric acidaemia
c) Chronic active hepatitis
d) Prolonged cholestasis
e) Sunflower cataracts

**251.** a) What is the likely diagnosis in this case?
b) Which two tests are likely to be most helpful in establishing a diagnosis?
c) Name three eye signs shown?

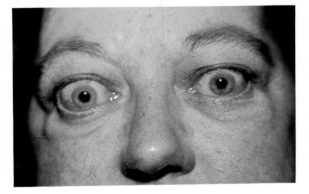

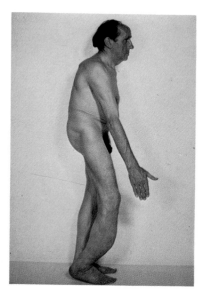

**252.** A most obvious abnormality is a very enlarged and bowed right tibia. Radiographs of the skull showed patchy bone accretion. What is the diagnosis?

**253.** Hyperkeratotic palmar lesions similar to these may be seen in which of the following?

   a) pompholyx
   b) ringworm of palms
   c) impetigo
   d) psoriasis
   e) secondary syphilis

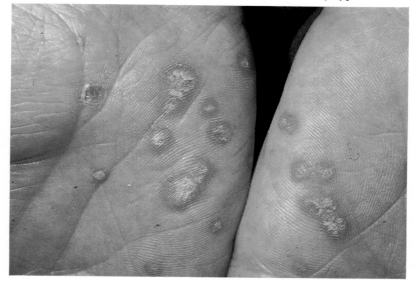

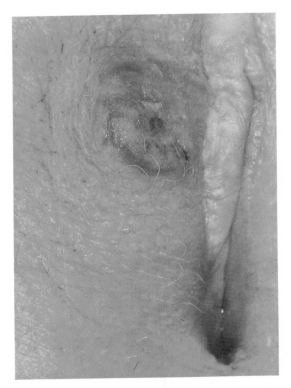

**254.** An elderly patient who complained of pruritus vulvae. What are the possible causes for the lesion found on examination?

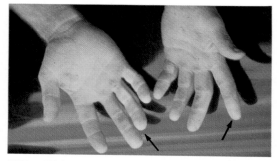

**255.** This patient developed pallor in the fingers during his work. What type of work did he participate in?

**256.** Infantile dermatitis of this pattern is commonly associated with which of the following?

a) urinary infection  b) asthma  c) myopia
d) hay fever  e) arthritis

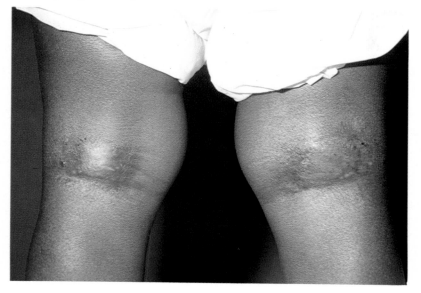

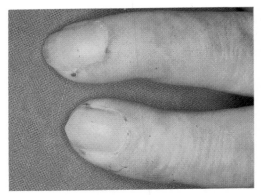

**257.** What is illustrated here and what are the underlying causes?

**258.** Gross enlargement, ulceration and intense pain of the tip of an index finger in a 68-year-old man who had had an abdominal operation 5 years previously. What is the diagnosis?

**259.** This 60-year-old man complained of a swelling below and in front of the lower lobe of the right ear. It had been present for several months. What is the differential diagnosis?

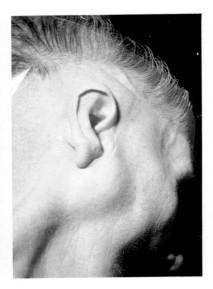

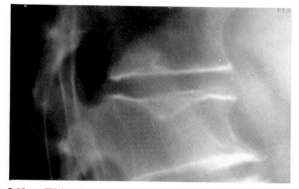

**260.** This 80-year-old female presented with backache. The X-ray of the dorsal spine shows?

    a) Paget's disease     d) Osteoporosis
    b) Multiple myeloma   e) Osteomalacia
    c) Schmorl's node

**261.** Such lesion could be the result of which of the following?

    a) Crush injury of the chest
    b) Diaphragmatic rupture
    c) Liver injury one day previously

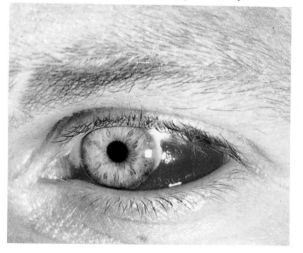

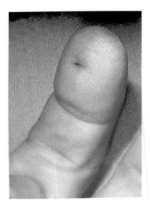

**262.** This patient had accidental injection of paint under high pressure when he used his left index finger pulp to clean the nozzle of a paint gun.
*Examination five hours after injury:* A very painful puncture wound.

a) What is the diagnosis?
b) What is the treatment?

**263.** Which of the following might be associated with this liver biopsy?

a) Sarcoidosis
b) Leptospirosis
c) Erythema Nodosum
d) Lymphocytic leukaemia
e) Leprosy

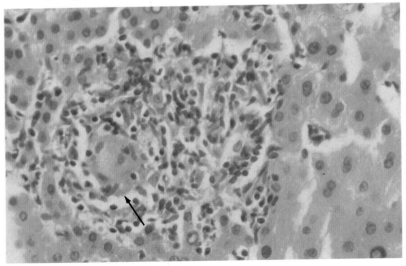

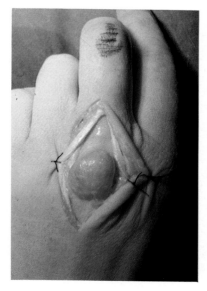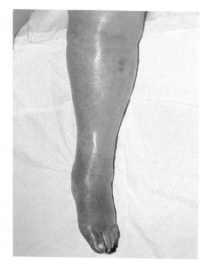

**264.** Cystic enlargement of an extensor tendon sheath on one finger of a young woman. What is the diagnosis?

**265.** A rapid painful swelling of the leg occurred in this lady and gangrene to the toes developed. What is the diagnosis and treatment?

**266.** What is this condition which causes severe throbbing pain?

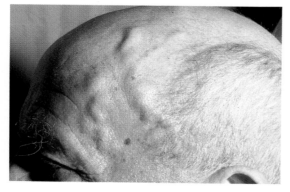

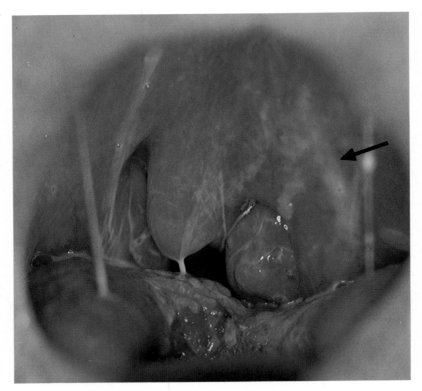

**267.** With which of the following may a quinsy (peri-tonsillar abscess) be very dangerous?

a) When associated with glandular fever
b) When it presents in childhood
c) When there is fresh bleeding
d) When it is bilateral

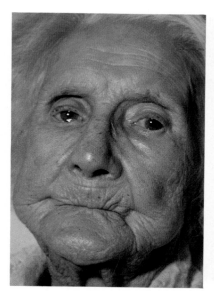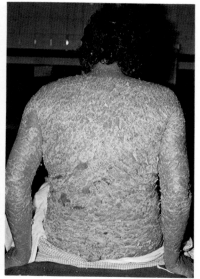

**268.** This 70-year-old lady was seen with jaundice and noted to have an enlarged gallbladder and liver. Note the jaundice only affects one eye! What diagnosis does that suggest?

**269.** Exfoliative erythroderma similar to this can occur in which of the following?

a) secondary syphilis
b) atopic dermatitis
c) lymphomas
d) psoriasis
e) drug reactions

**270.** Which findings might be included in the patient with this coeliac angiogram?

a) Haemoptysis
b) Hypoglycocaemia
c) Positive serum hepatitis B surface antigen test
d) Positive serum carcino embryonic antigen test
e) An abdominal bruit

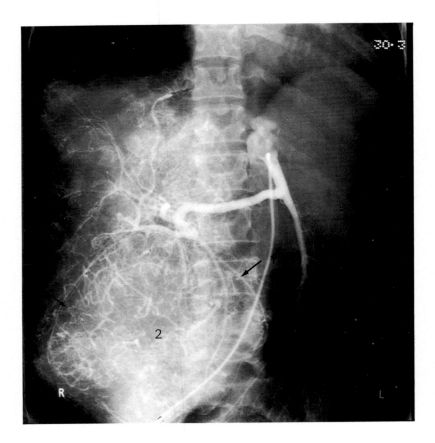

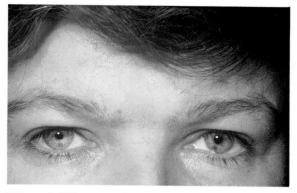

271.  a) What eye signs are depicted?
      b) Can they form part of a syndrome? If so, which one?
      c) Name one complication of this syndrome?
      d) Does it occur in all gene carriers?
      e) What are the risks to his offspring?

272.  This tonsillar membrane is characteristic of which of the
      following?

      a) Diphtheria  b) A fungal infection
      c) Infectious mononeucleosis  d) Vincent's angina

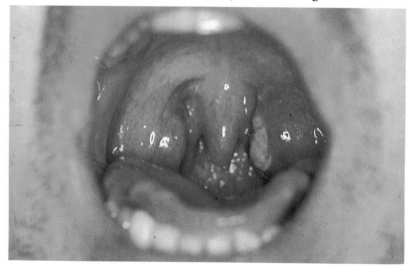

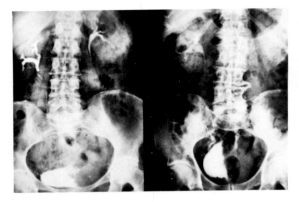

**273.**
Two IVUs.
Both show bladder
filling defects.
What are the
differences?

**274.** a) What is the clinical
diagnosis?
b) In view of the sex of
this patient, what is
the most likely
cause?

**275.** Lesions at sites of
injury or pressure are
typically seen in which
of the following?

a) eczema
b) psoriasis
c) lichen planus

d) viral warts
e) seborrhoeic
warts

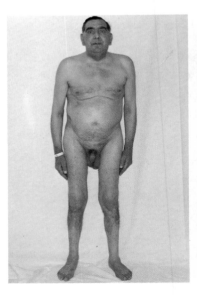

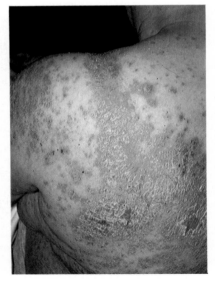

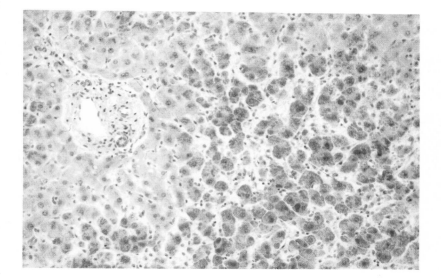

**276.** This needle liver biopsy came from a woman 4 weeks after delivery of a stillborn baby. Which of the following might have been included in the clinical picture and investigations?

a) Persistent vomiting
b) Low serum uric acid level
c) Blood film showing nucleated red blood cells
d) Coma
e) Itching during pregnancy

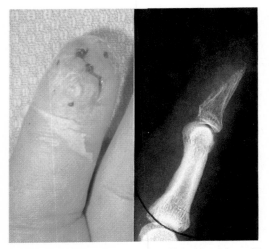

**277.** *History:* This patient lived by himself on an island. One week after a minor puncture wound from a splinter he developed throbbing pain in the pulp. Over the next three weeks he treated himself weekly by stabbing the pulp. On three different occasions he released pus and was relieved temporarily of pain. He presented six weeks later with pain and discharge from his finger tip.
*Examination:* Tenderness and swelling of the pulp. Pus drainage from each of the sinuses.

a) What is the differential diagnosis?
b) What investigations?
c) What is the treatment?

**279.** This young girl was referred with a swelling in the left side of the neck. It had gradually increased in size over three weeks at first not painful but gradually becoming so. A fluctuant swelling was noted without oedema associated with the redness. What was the probable diagnosis and management?

**278.** What is this patient's complaint? Why the oedema? What is the underlying cause?

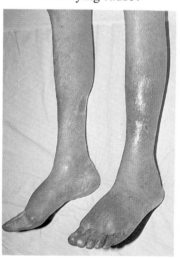

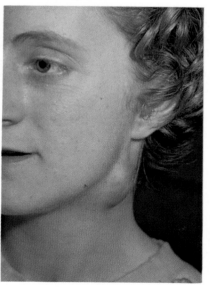

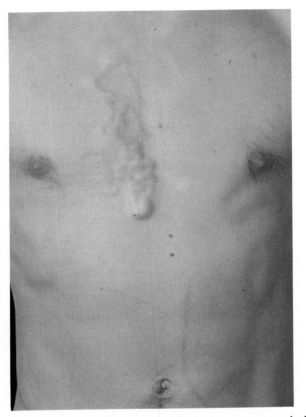

**280.** Which of the following statements are probably true in this patient?

    a) The origin of the abdominal wall veins is the right portal vein

    b) The condition has been termed caput medusae

    c) The patient may have oesophageal varices

    d) The blood flow in the veins is towards the umbilicus

    e) The patient usually has ankle oedema

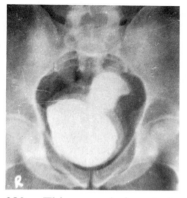

**281.** Bladder film of IVU. What abnormality?

**282.** This young lady noted the development of this lesion in childhood. It grew slowly to the present size. What changes would cause concern and require surgery?

**283.** What common condition is illustrated? What complication may occur causing severe pain and distress, and what is the best treatment?

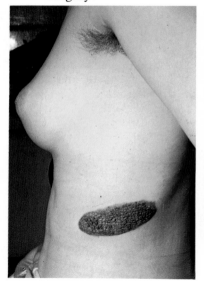

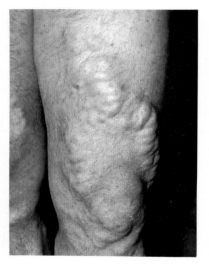

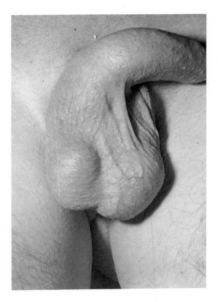

**284.** A 30-year-old man noticed in the bath, a swelling in the left side of the scrotum. There was only a slight discomfort associated with it and he therefore delayed being seen for 2 months. What investigations should be carried out to establish the diagnosis?

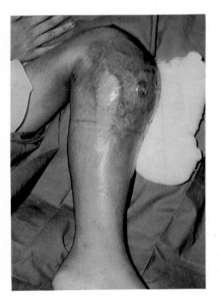

**285.** Enlargement and intense pain just below the knee of a 26-year-old man. There was overlying ulceration of the skin and increased vascularity. What is the diagnosis?

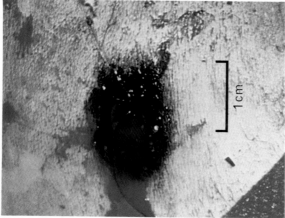

1 cm

**286.** From what distance did this gunshot wound occur?

    a) Fired point-blank
    b) Fired from close range
    c) Fired from a 3 metres distance

**287.** In what way is the cornea abnormal and what are the possible causes?

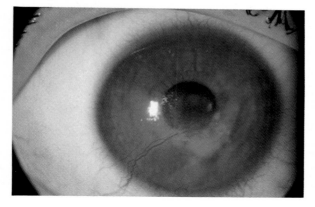

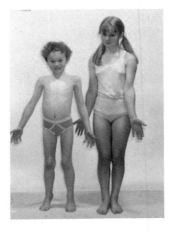

**288.** a) The boy has Duchenne muscular dystrophy — how is this inherited?
b) If mother had an affected brother what is the risk of his sister (in the photograph) being a carrier?
c) What tests would you do on this girl?

**289.** a) What is this condition?
b) What may precipitate it?
c) What is the treatment?

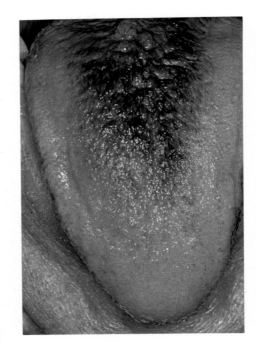

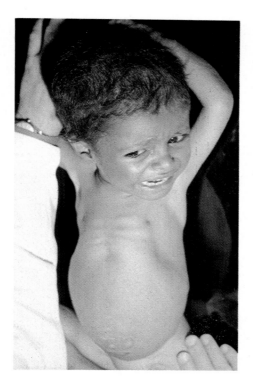

**290.** Whose name is associated with this groove of the lower ribs?

**291.** The ulceration of this limb has persisted for several years. What are the possible causes and problems of management?

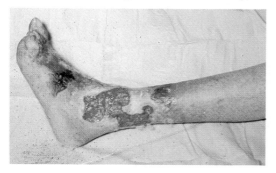

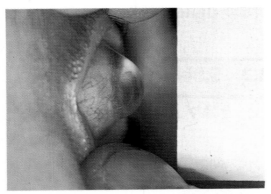

**292.** What is the cause of the abnormal profile of the cornea?

**293.** a) What is the diagnosis?
b) Name the three most common causative organisms of this entity.

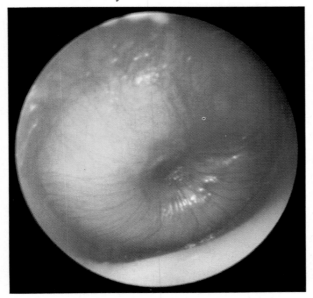

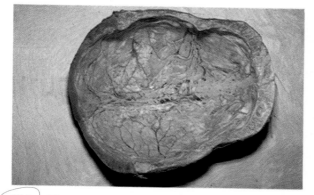

**294.** The skull of a deaf patient who had died suddenly following a fractured femur showed thickening of the bones, particularly in the frontal region. Which of the following is the most likely diagnosis?

a) Hyperostosis Frontalis Interna
b) Sturge Weber syndrome
c) Kartageners syndrome
d) Paget's Disease
e) Fluorosis

**295.** Filling defect in bladder — What is the cause?

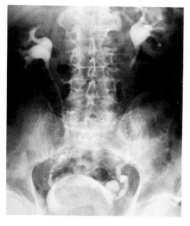

**296.** What abnormality?

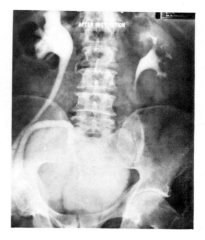

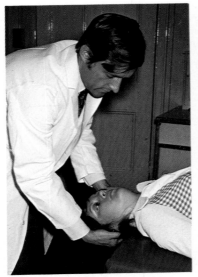

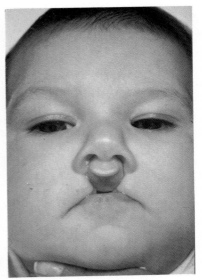

**297.** This test may be
diagnostic for which of
the following?

a) Cervical spine
   osteoarthritis
b) Benign paroxismal
   positional vertigo
c) A perilymph fistula
d) Erosion of the lateral
   semi-circular canal

**298.** a) What abnormal
       physical signs are
       shown here?
   b) What is the
       diagnosis?
   c) What is the
       inheritance pattern?

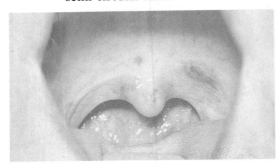

**299.** a) What is this
       abnormality?
   b) Where is
       the lesion?
   c) What are
       the common
       causes?

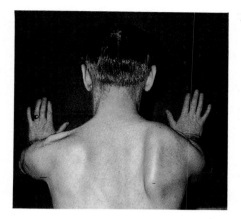

**300.** a) What is this condition called?
b) Where is it due to?
c) What are the common causes?

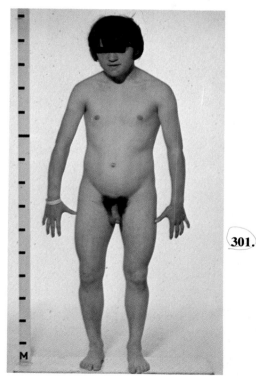

**301.** a) What is the diagnosis in this 8-year-old boy?
b) Will the bone age be advanced or retarded?
c) If the blood pressure is $160/100$ what is the most likely diagnosis?

**302.** An unusual tumour with a poor prognosis. What would be
the most appropriate treatment?

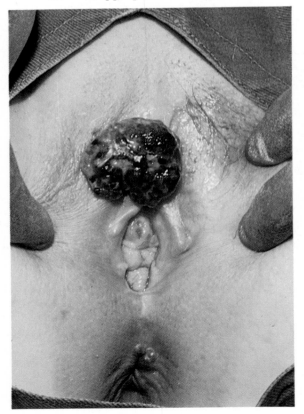

**303.** This lesion developed as a papule on the nose and increased in size over 2 months when it broke down to form an ulcerated lesion. There was no enlargement of lymphatic glands. What is the likely diagnosis and how might it be treated?

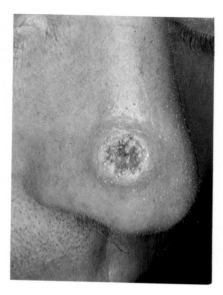

**304.** This well-defined facial erythema is probably due to which of the following?

a) Maxillary sinusitis
b) Erysipelas
c) Rosacea
d) Dental infection

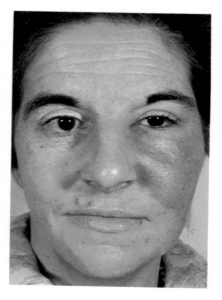

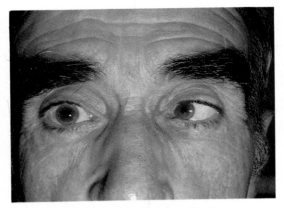

**305.** a) What is this abnormality?
   b) What other signs would you expect to find?
   c) What are the two most common causes?

**306.** This is the oral presentation of what is often thought of as a skin disease.

   a) What might it be?
   b) What form of skin lesions may be associated with it?
   c) What may precipitate the condition?

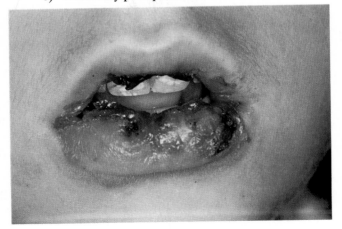

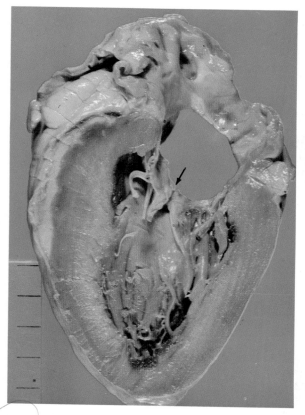

**307.**  a) Name the defect and its type.
b) State its anatomical relationship into the fossa ovalis.
c) Comment on the malformation arrowed.

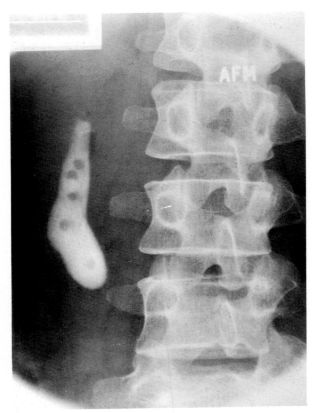

**308.** The appearances in this oral cholecystogram might be associated with which of the following?

    a) High biliary phospholipid concentration.
    b) Suitability for ursodeoxycholic acid therapy.
    c) Chronic pancreatitis.
    d) Oral contraceptive (birth control) ills.
    e) Cholestatic jaundice.

**309.**
a) What is the diagnosis?
b) What do you call the lesion on his chin and those on his forehead?
c) What are the risks to his offspring if neither of his parents are affected?
d) How would you examine his sister who seems unaffected and wants to have children?

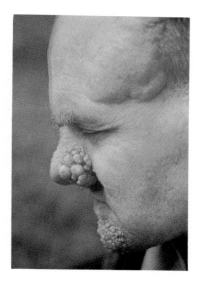

**310.**
a) What is the diagnosis?
b) What abnormalities are visible?
c) What other abnormalities are commonly found on examination?
d) What are the most dangerous features of the condition?

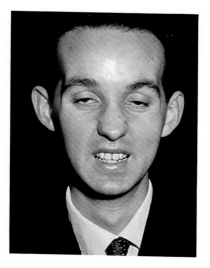

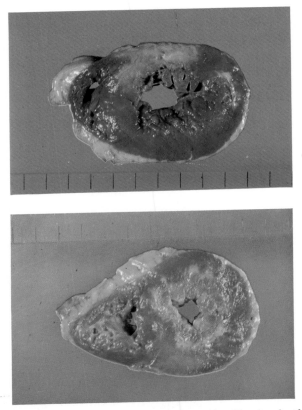

**311.** a) Name the condition that is affecting both hearts.
b) Name the two different types and comment on their anatomical localisation and the cause for this.

**312.** This 70-year-old female patient presented with lethargy, immobility, confusion and constipation. What are the likely causes?

a) Abdominal aortic aneurysm
b) Hypothyroidism
c) Hypothermia
d) Pemphigus
e) Advanced cerebrovascular disease

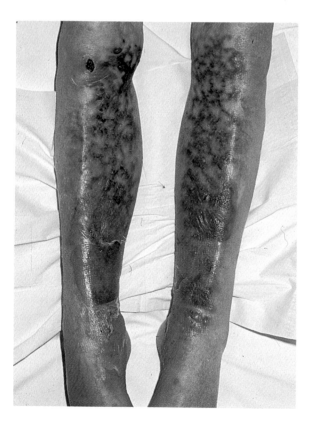

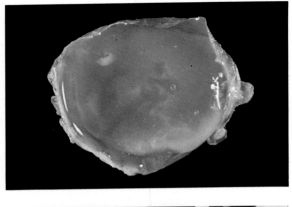

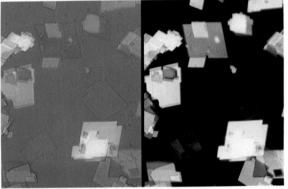

**313.** What is the nature of these crystals from a branchial cleft cyst?
List five pathological lesions other than cysts in which this crystalline material or its esters commonly accumulate.

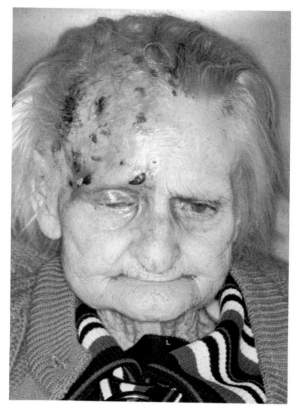

**314.** Which of the following conditions may occur as a
complication of the disorder shown above?

    a) Ramsay-Hunt syndrome
    b) Cataracts
    c) Proptosis
    d) Encephalitis
    e) Depression

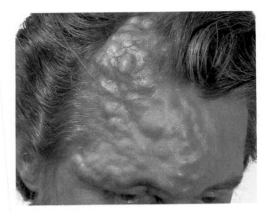

**315.** This was present in the young man for eight years or more. What is the diagnosis?

**316.** a) What abnormalities are visible?
b) What are the likely causes?
c) How would you distinguish between them?

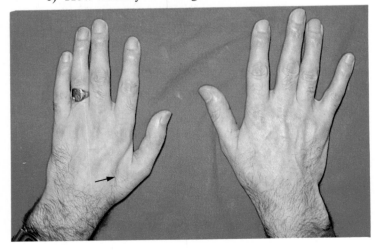

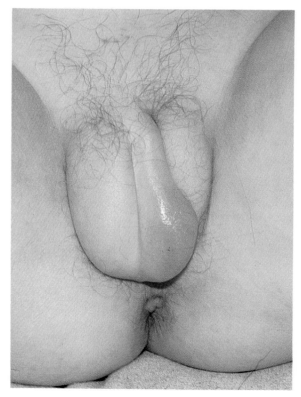

**317.** A rather unusual case of oedema of the vulva. Can you
suggest some causes?

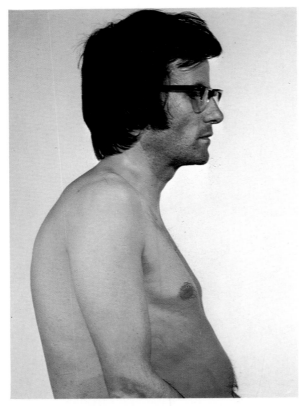

**318.** Kypohosis and spinal crush fractures associated with abdominal enlargement in a 32-year-old man. Which of the following is likely to be the cause?

 a)  Cushing's Syndrome
 b)  High alcohol intake
 c)  Chronic cirrhosis
 d)  Diabetes mellitus
 e)  Primary thyrotoxicosis

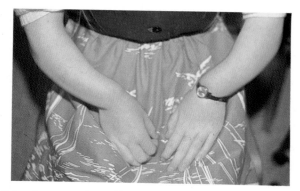

319. a) What do this photograph and X-ray show?
    b) What is the diagnosis?
    c) What are the other features and inheritance of this
       syndrome?

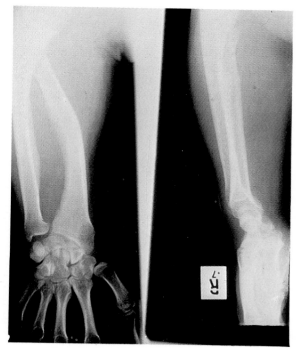

195

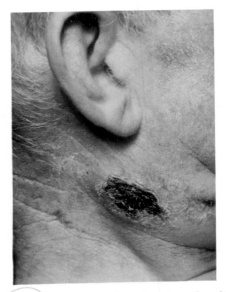

**320.** A farm worker developed an itchy swelling on the right side of the neck. It gradually increased in size over the next few days and appeared as a reddish black swelling with a ring of small vesicles round it. Lymph nodes were enlarged. The swelling broke down and a black slough appeared. He was referred as a possible carbuncle. How would the proper diagnosis be established?

**321.**

a) What is the cause of this pannus?

b) What other condition can cause pannus?

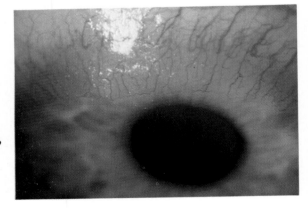

**322.** What conclusion can be made from this patient? What could be a possible cause? Could there be an insect vector?

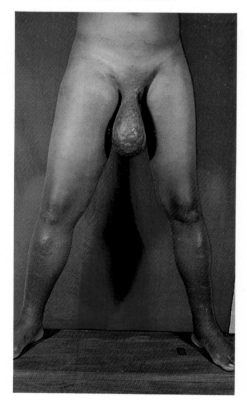

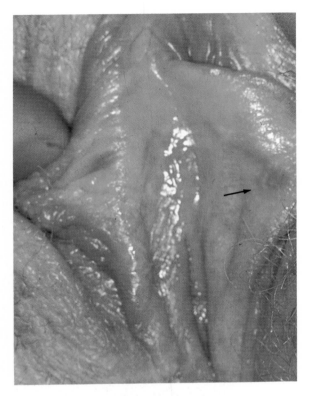

**323.**  a) This patient complained of pruritus vulvae. Can you
suggest a possible cause?
b) The patient was also noted to have similar small lesions
on the lips. What condition is associated with cyclical
oral and vulval ulcers?

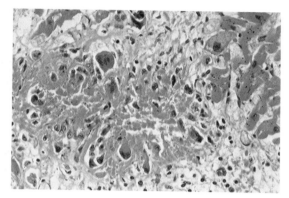

**324.**  a) Name the lesion?
    b) In which disease does it occur?
    c) Describe the appearance of the lesion and its cell
       constituence

**325.**  a) What is this condition, and where is the lesion?
    b) What are the two most common causes?

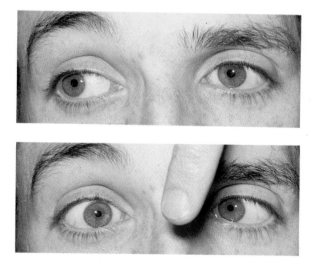

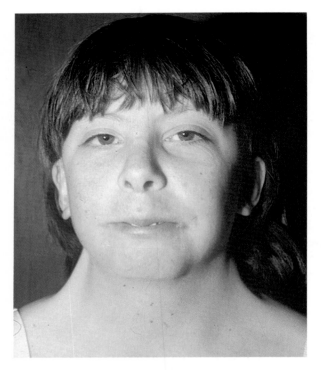

**326.**  a) What is the most likely diagnosis here?
b) What are the other clinical features of this syndrome?
c) How would you confirm the diagnosis and what would you expect to find?

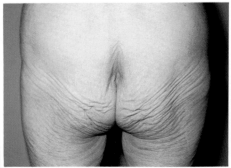

**327.**  a) What does this picture show?
b) What is the characteristic symptom in such patients?
c) What are the main causes?

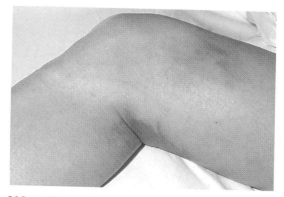

**328.** This patient was aware of a throbbing mass behind the knee. Increase of pain was associated with bruising due to what?

**329.** A 45-year-old labourer had painful paraesthesiae in his left hand waking him at night. During the day he noticed weakness and clumsiness of his left hand.
*Examination:* Lack of work staining of his left thumb, index, and middle fingers. Thenar muscle wasting and lack of opposition.

   a) What is the differential diagnosis?
   b) What is the treatment?

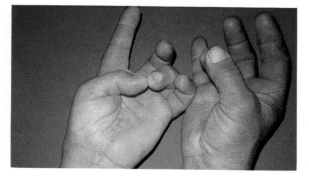

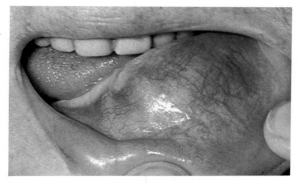

330. A 39-year-old patient with recurrent bone pain and with difficulty in the occlusion of his lower jaw was found to have a large swelling protruding from his mandible. Which of the following is the most likely diagnosis?
a) An epulis
b) An adamantinoma
c) A dental cyst
d) An osteoclastoma
e) Chronic osteomyelitis

331. This barium enema study in a patient with periodical, colicky abdominal pain suggests which of the following?
a) Cancer of the splenic flexure
b) Possible post-traumatic colothorax
c) Pneumatosis cystoides intestinalis

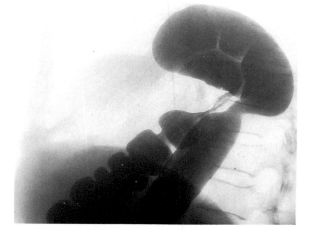

**332.** The diagnosis is relatively easy, but can you suggest some causes, and the usual symptoms?

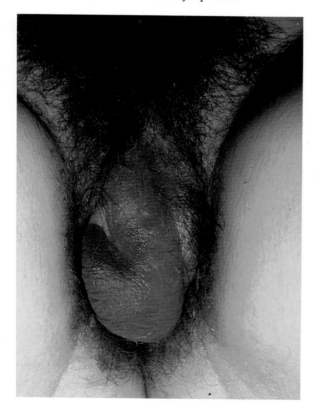

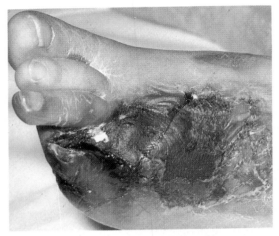

**333.** In what type of patient would you expect to see this type of moist gangrene?

**334.** a) Name the condition affecting this mitral valve.
　　　b) Describe the appearance of the valve.
　　　c) Describe the pathology of the valve.
　　　d) Name two complications of this condition.

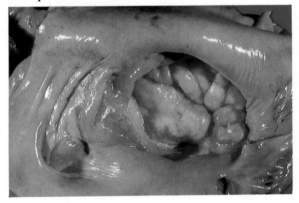

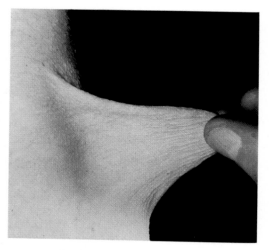

**335.** What does this demonstrate in the skin? What extremely serious arterial condition may develop in this patient?

**336.** a) This patient is diabetic. What is the likely diagnosis?
b) How would you avoid this condition?

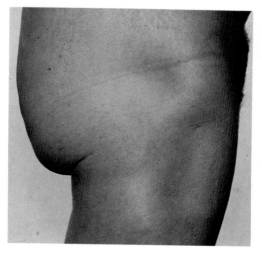

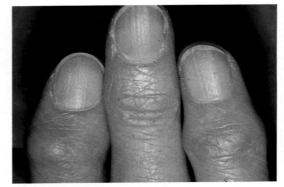

**337.** The distal fingers of a middle-aged man. Enlargement has gradually developed over the years and there is no associated history of trauma or other disease. What is the diagnosis?

**338.** a) Describe the abnormality.
b) Discuss the differential diagnosis.
c) How do you confirm the diagnosis?
d) What is the treatment?

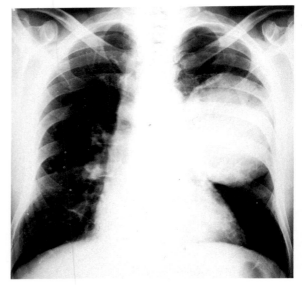

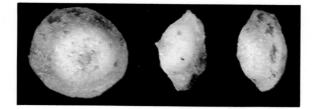

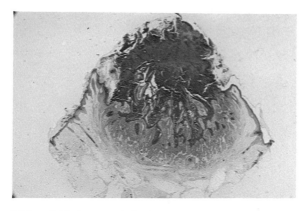

**339.** This keratotic lesion from the face has reached this size in three months. Are the following statements true of false?

a) This is a self-healing keratoacanthoma

b) Histologically it is easily distinguishable from a well-differentiated squamous cell carcinoma

c) It represents a disturbance of normal hair growth cycle

d) Shaving off the lesion flush with the skin is an acceptable form of treatment

e) Lymph node metastases never occur

f) It is a well recognised pre-cancerous condition

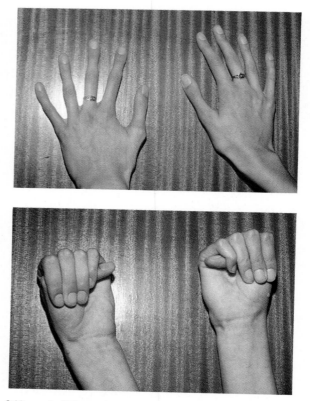

**340.** a) What abnormality is shown here?
b) What sign is demonstrated in the lower picture?
c) In which syndromes is this abnormality found?

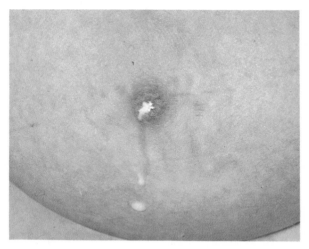

**341.** Galactorrhoea is lactation in the absence of an appropriate physiological stimulus.

    a) Is galactorrhoea always associated with an elevated serum prolactin level?

    b) Name three drugs which cause galactorrhoea?

    c) Which thyroid complaint may be associated with galactorrhoea?

**342.** This swelling behind the angle of the left jaw grew gradually without pain or redness. It could move slightly from side to side but not vertically. Pulsation was felt but not obviously expansile. What is the diagnosis?

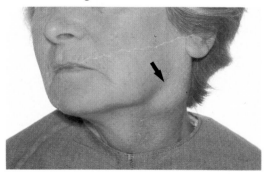

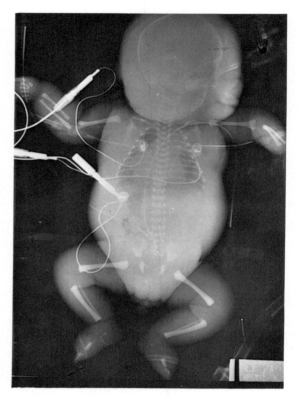

**343.** a) What is this?
b) Give two causes other than blood group anomalies?

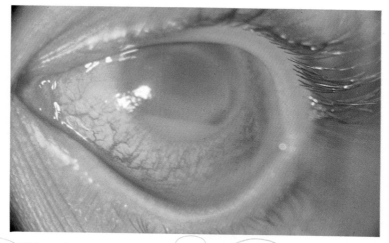

**344.** This patient presented with oral and genital ulceration as well as ocular inflammation.

    a) Name the syndrome characterised by this clinical triad?

    b) Name the ocular abnormality shown in the illustration?

    c) Thrombophlebitis is a known complication of the syndrome: what additional ocular abnormality might be seen on examination of the fundus?

**345.** A man of 40 years presented with gangrene of the toes and marked pain. He smoked 40 cigarettes a day. Popliteal pulses were palpable. What was the diagnosis?

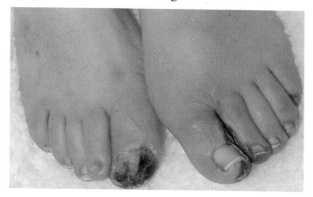

**346.** a) What is the diagnosis?
 b) Name three characteristic clinical features
 c) Name three diseases associated with this condition

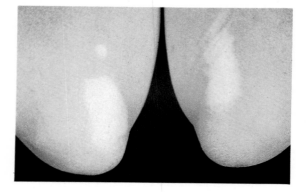

**347.** a) What is this condition?
 b) What are the common causes?
 c) What are the complications?
 d) What is the main treatment?

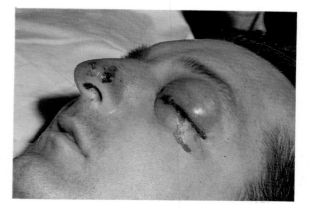

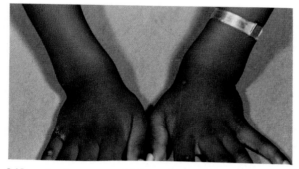

**348.** A nine-year-old Jamaican girl presented with painful symmetrical swollen wrists. Which of the following would be the likely causes of this condition?

a) Stills Disease (Juvenile Rheumatoid Arthritis)
b) Nutritional rickets
c) Renal tubular rickets
d) Osteomyelitis
e) Osteogenesis imperfecta

**349.** This 56-year-old man developed a rapid swelling of the left arm after painting a ceiling. The arm became bluish-red. What is the diagnosis and why has the swelling developed?

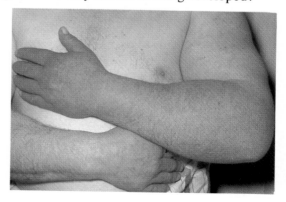

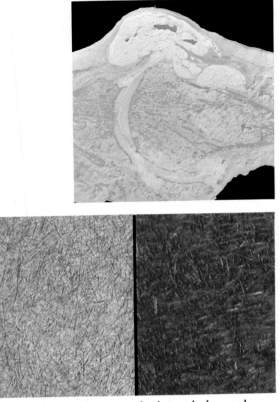

**350.** What name is given to a swelling over the interphalangeal joint of the big toe in a patient with gout? Are the following statements true of false?

Crystals of sodium bi-urate
a) are strongly negatively birefringent
b) are usually needle-shaped
c) are insoluble in ordinary formalin containing fixative
d) may be deposited in bursae
e) may be deposited in bone and marrow
f) are demonstrable in synovial fluid within leucocytes and free in the fluid during attacks of gouty arthritis
g) react with nitric acid and ammonium hydroxide to give a purple colour (murexide test)

**351.** Why do blood vessels grow into the deep cornea of a patient wearing soft hydrophilic contact lenses?

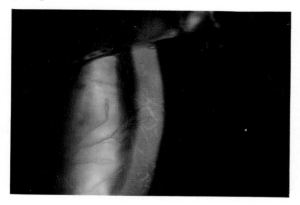

**352.** a) What does this slide show?
b) What other signs would you look for?
c) What is the condition with which this disease is often confused?

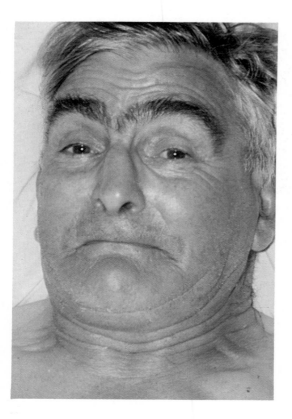

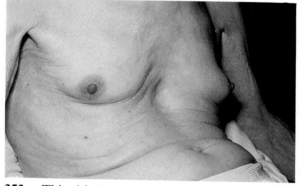

**353.** This elderly man has gynaecomastia. Which of the following is likely to be the underlying disorder?

a) Motor neurone disease
b) Acromegaly
c) Cardiac amyloidosis
d) Carcinoma bronchus
e) Polymyalgia rheumatica

**354.**
a) Describe the abnormality shown in the illustration?
b) What are the most likely diagnoses?
c) What is the commonest ocular abnormality associated with the disorder illustrated?

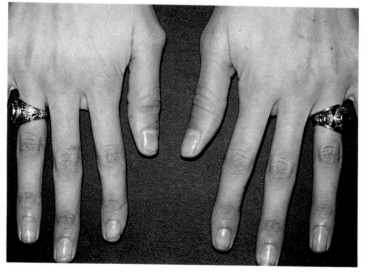

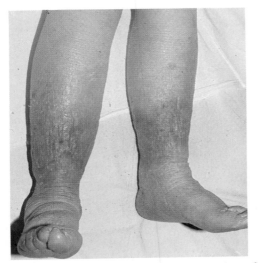

**355.** The swelling of both legs and the cellulitis appeared in this patient in her early forties. Now nearly 50 years old, the swelling and cellulitis have steadily progressed. What is the diagnosis and treatment?

**356.** Which of the following is true of incontineutia pigmenta?
   a) is inherited as an X linked recessive
   b) affects only the skin
   c) is commonly found on the scalp
   d) may display a linear distribution
   e) has skin lesions which classically evolve

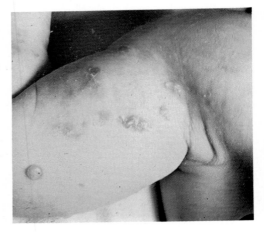

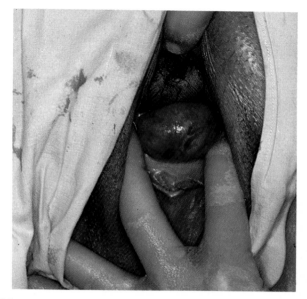

**357.** What two objects are visible in the vagina?

**358.** Which of the following statements are true of the islets of Langerhans in the pancreas?

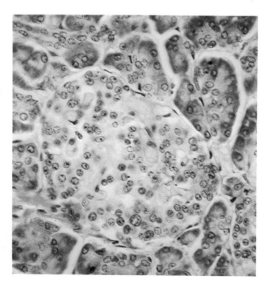

    a) They secrete pepsin
    b) They secrete insulin
    c) They secrete glucagon
    d) They contain serous acini
    e) They contain alpha, beta and delta cells

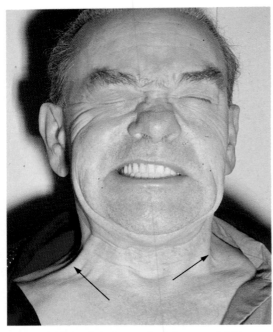

**359.** a) What is this abnormality?
b) What would you test next?
c) Why?

**360.** This is the chest of a 16-year-old boy.

a) What is the likely diagnosis?
b) Would the prolactin level be significantly raised?
c) What advice would you give?

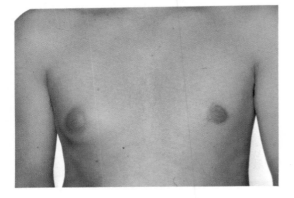

**361.** a) What is this?
b) Give three stigmata demonstrated in this picture?

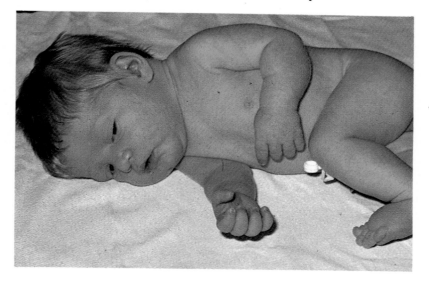

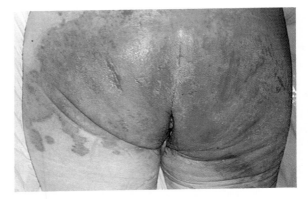

**362.** This skin lesion on the back of an elderly female patient may be due to?

a) Dermatitis herpetiformis    d) Faecal incontinence
b) Urinary incontinence    e) Vasculitis
c) Erythema multiforme

**363.** This patient had crushed several vertebrae in her spine and her hands showed skin changes which could be associated with which of the following?

a) Senile purpura and osteoporosis
b) Long term steroid therapy for rheumatoid arthritis
c) Mastocytosis  d) Chronic alcoholism  e) Malnutrition

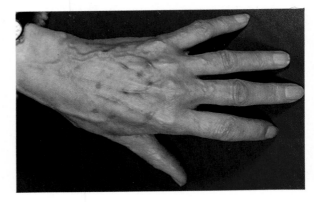

**364.** What is this and how is it treated?

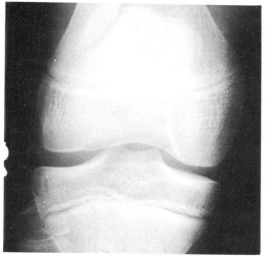

**365.** This patient has a prolonged grip and handshake.

a) Name the ocular abnormality shown in the illustration.
b) Of what condition is it pathognomic?

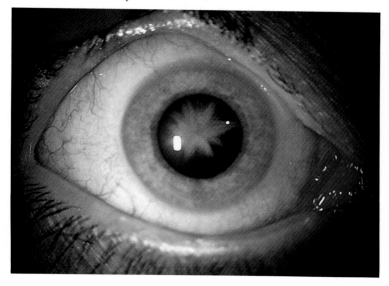

**366.** Which of these statements apply to the wall of a bronchiole?

    a) The lining epithelium is simple ciliated columnar
    b) The lining is simple columnar
    c) Hyaline cartilage is absent from the wall
    d) Mucoserous glands are absent from the wall
    e) There is an incomplete cuff of smooth muscle
    f) There is a complete cuff of smooth muscle

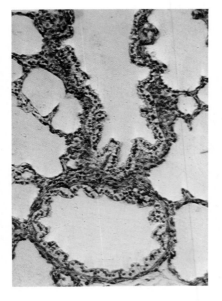

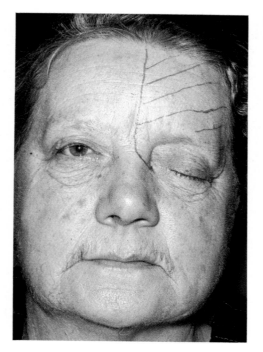

**367.** a) What is this condition?

b) What abnormalities would you expect to find if the left eye was opened, and what is the most likely cause?

**368.** If this patient had amenorrhoea, what are the possible causes? What tests are indicated if infertility is also a symptom? What drug might be effective for several of the causes?

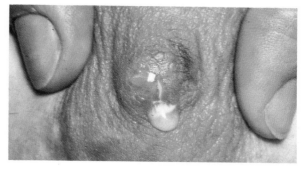

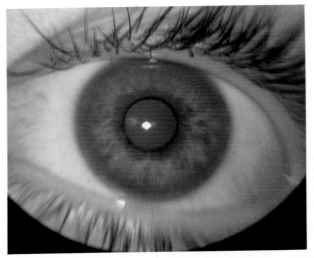

**369.** This patient presented with involuntary movements of the limbs. Hepatomegaly was also present, as well as the ocular abnormality shown in the illustration.

   a) Name this ocular abnormality. How does it arise?
   b) What is the diagnosis?
   c) What other ocular abnormality may occur in this disease?

**370.** This elderly man presented with a fractured femur and this skin condition. Which of the following is a likely cause of his bone disease?

   a) Osteoporosis       d) Hyperparathyroidism
   b) Paget's Disease     e) Metastic carcinoma of the
   c) Osteomalacia          oesophagus

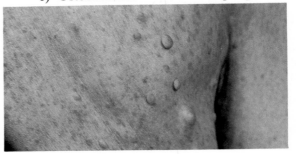

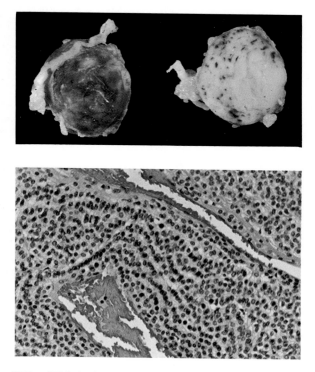

**371.** This lesion on the fifth finger of a 70-year-old man was associated with paroxysms of pain. What is the likely diagnosis?

Indicate briefly
a) Its origin
b) The sex incidence
c) Site
d) Principal histological components

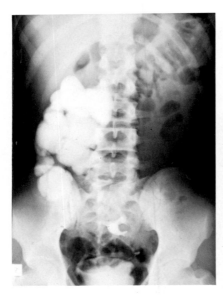 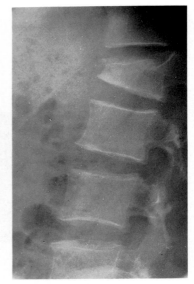

**372.** How many and what congenital abnormalities are present?

**373.** a) What is the differential diagnosis?
b) What neurological signs might appear with an acute lesion of this sort?
c) What is the management?

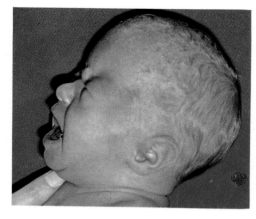

**374.**

Which of the following are features of Crouzon's syndrome?

a) Autosomal recessive inheritance
b) Premature fusion of the lambdoid sutures
c) Micrognathia
d) Blindness in untreated cases
e) Hypertelorism

**375.** This skin lesion from the medial aspect of calf is hard and raised with cream-coloured patchy brownish cut surface. When treated with Sudan IV (middle) much of the lesion stains red and with Perls' stain a strong Prussian Blue reaction is obtained:

a) What is the lesion?
b) What constituent reacts (i)   with Sudan IV?
                         (ii)   with Perls' reagent?
c) If the pathologist reports that the lesion has been incompletely excised is it essential to remove the residual lesional tissue?
d) What is known about the aetiology of this lesion?

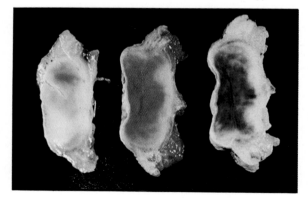

**376.** This woman, aged 40 years, presented with haematemesis. On examination she was found to have yellow plaque-like lesions in her neck, antecubital fossae and groins, as well as abnormalities of the retina.

a) Name and describe the retinal abnormalities shown in the illustration.

b) What visual symptoms may occur?

c) Name the syndrome and review its characteristic features?

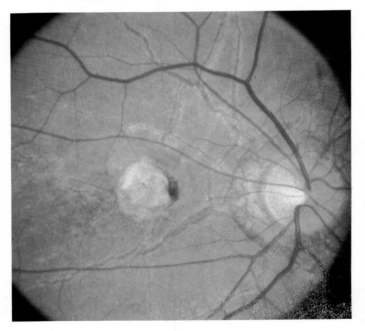

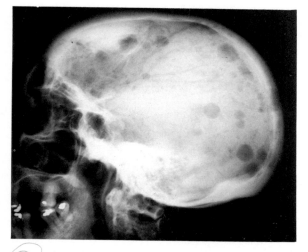

**377.** a) What is the abnormal appearance? b) Suggest a diagnosis c) Describe symptoms and signs d) How do you confirm the diagnosis? e) What is the treatment?

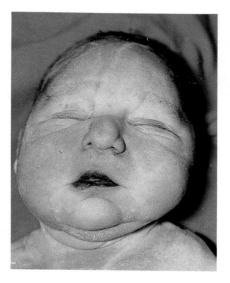

**378.** Which of the following are commonly found in Potter's syndrome?

    a) Hypotelorism
    b) Limb deformities
    c) Hydrocephalus
    d) Hydramnios
    e) Megapenis

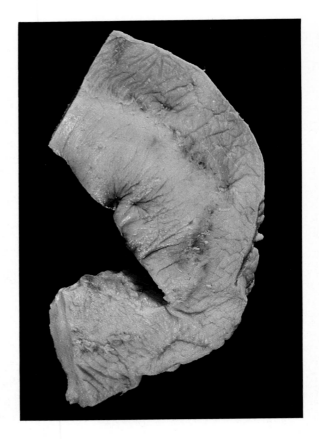

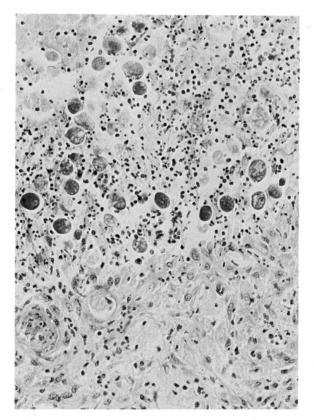

**379.** Given the history and the histological preparation in which PAS positive structures are seen amongst the granulation tissue and exudate in the undermined edge of the abdominal wound, what is the diagnosis?
List four investigations which would enable you to confirm this.

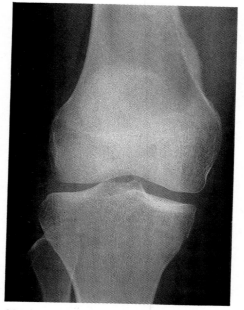

**380.** This patient complained of knee pain after netball. Why is "rest" the wrong treatment?

**381.** A young patient with polyuria for several months complained of sore, gritty eyes, the conjunctiva looks inflamed. The patient could be suffering from which of the following?

a) Hyperparathyroidism b) Sarcoidosis c) Chronic renal failure d) Reiters Syndrome e) Amino Aciduria

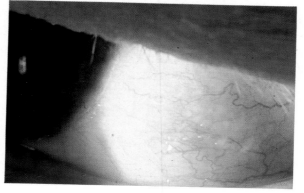

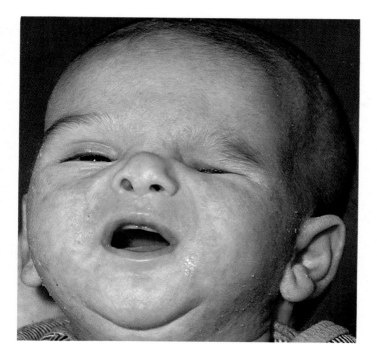

**382.** a) What does this picture demonstrate?
   b) In what syndrome may this be found?

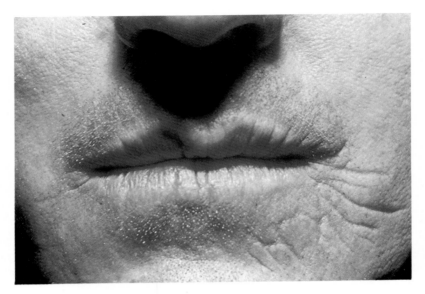

**383.** What is shown in this picture?

**384.** a) Describe what you see? b) What does the needle point to? c) What were the patient's symptoms and signs? d) How was the diagnosis confirmed? e) What is the treatment?

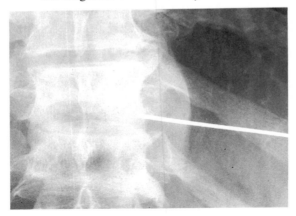

**385.** Which of the
following are
features of this
syndrome?

a) Hypercalcaemia
b) Irritability
c) Bone fragility
d) Sex linked
   inheritance
e) Metaphyseal
   flaring

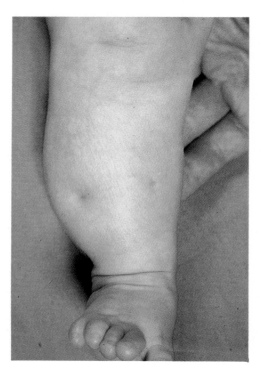

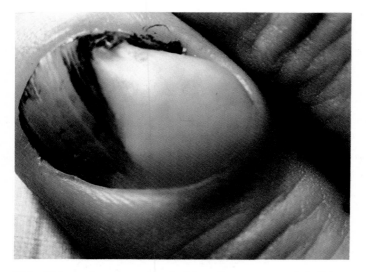

**386.** This patient presented with epilepsy, mental deficiency and adenoma sebaceum.

   a) Describe the lesion shown in the illustration; it is a pathognomic feature of the disease.

   b) What is the name of the disease?

   c) What abnormality may be found on examination of the ocular fundus?

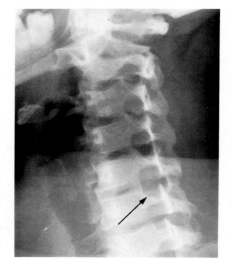

**387.** a) What abnormality does this X-ray show?

   b) What is the probable cause?

   c) What signs would you expect to find?

238

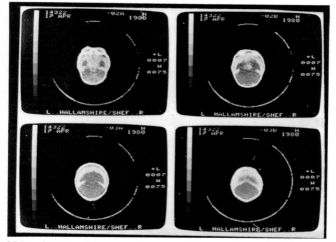

**388.** a) Describe two abnormalities on this CAT scan.
    b) What is the most likely diagnosis?

**389.** This patient presented with dusky pink irritant plaques on
the glans penis; buccal findings are depicted in the
photograph. What is the diagnosis?

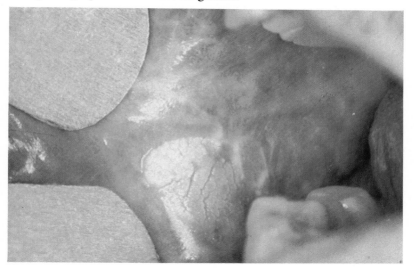

**390.** A 20-year-old girl with intense pain in the right ankle. There was no local signs of abnormality. The plain radiograph was normal, but the tomographs shows a lesion in the neck of the talus.

**391.** This infant's parents had generalised irritant skin rashes.

a) What is the most likely diagnosis?
b) What other conditions should be excluded?

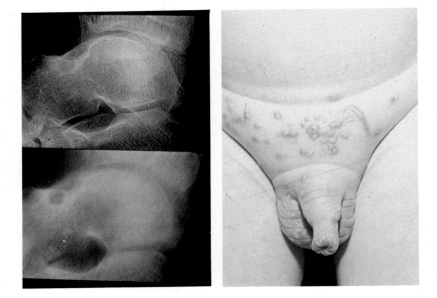

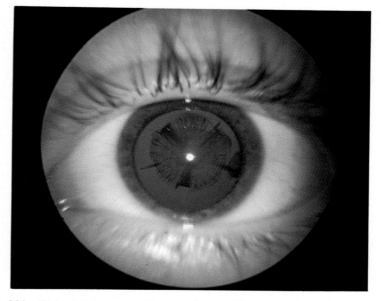

**392.** This child is mentally retarded and has an enlarged liver.

    a) Describe the ocular abnormality shown in the illustration.
    b) What is the most likely diagnosis?

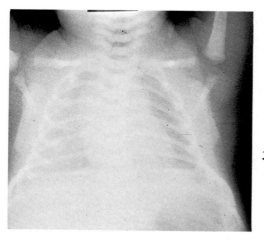

**393.** a) What does this radiograph demonstrate?
      b) What is the most common aetiology?

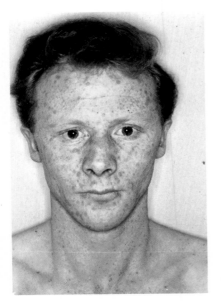

**394.** a) What does the appearance of this writing suggest?
b) Three points in the history might help to confirm the diagnosis. What are they?
c) What is the drug of choice?

**395.** The rash depicted was non-irritant; the only other abnormality found was generalised moderate lymph gland enlargement.
What investigations are likely to help diagnosis?

**396.** a) What is this?
b) What is the aetiology?
c) At what level is the primary lesion?

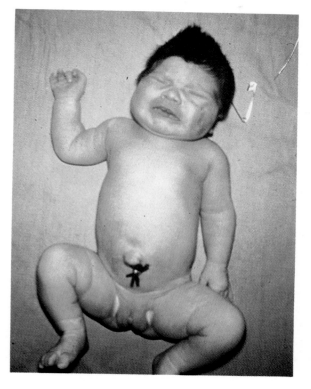

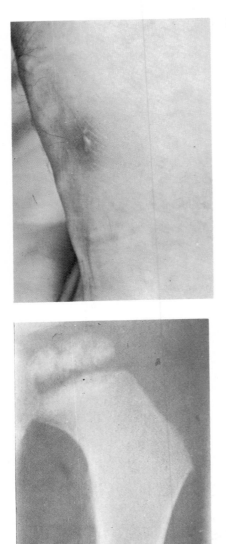

**397.** This vesico-pustule was one of several found on a nineteen-year-old woman with salpingitis. What is the likely diagnosis and why is this only likely to be established when such manifestations occur?

**398.** The condition shown here may be seen in which of the following?

a) Maternal warfarin administration.
b) Congenital dislocation of the hip.
c) Spina bifida.
d) Hypothyroidism.
e) Pierre Robin syndrome.

**399.** This patient had "inflamed eyes and joints" in childhood.

    a) What abnormality is shown in the photograph?
    b) What is the aetiology?

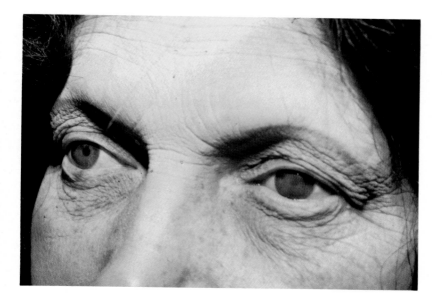

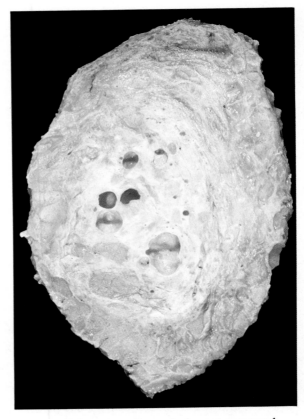

**400.** This is a photograph of the cut surface of a breast removed from a forty-seven-year-old patient complaining of a tender mass and a discharge from the nipple. What is the name given to this condition? Are the following statements true or false?

This pathological lesion
a) is commoner in the nullipara than multipara.
b) is common after the menopause.
c) is usually unilateral.
d) is precancerous.

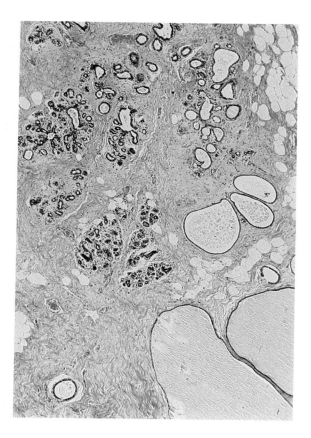

e) in adolescence may be associated with endometrial
hyperplasia.
f) may present with curiously coloured (green or blue)
discharge from the nipple.

# Answers

1. Epanutin (phenytoin).
   **ofd**

2. Keratoconus — a non inflammatory stromal (collagen) degeneration affecting 1 in 10,000 individuals to variable degrees and often associated with atopy.
   **col**

3. Yes to c). a) and b) possibly.
   **bd**

4. Diabetic nephropathy with heavy proteinuria and hypertension.
   **di**

5. Adult *Loa loa* in the eye. The movement of the adult worm under the conjunctiva gives rise to considerable irritation and congestion.
   **tmp**

6. Could have sustained chest injury.
   **chtr**

7. *Troisier's sign* Enlargement of the gland in the left supraclavicular fossa in a patient with carcinoma of the stomach. Drainage occurs straight upwards and the left supraclavicular fossa should always be palpated when carcinoma of the stomach is suspected, even though no mass is felt in the stomach. *(Charles Emile Troisier, 1849-1919.)*
   **psgm**

8. *Fasciola hepatica* (liver fluke) is only infectious to man by ingestion of larval stages encysted on water plants.
   **tmp**

9. They usually indicate a bad prognosis.
   **rh**

10. Early diabetic retinopathy.

If this is the presenting symptom then clearly systemic manifestations must receive urgent attention but advanced untreated diabetic retinopathy is now a common cause of blindness so early specialist assessment is vital.
**od**

11. Riboflavin.
    **nd**

12. Infantile kala-azar. Children present with irregular fever, anaemia, a moderately enlarged, non-tender liver, and a greatly enlarged firm spleen.
    **tmp**

13. Ochronosis — bluish black discoloration of cartilage in those suffering from alkaptonuria.
    **rh**

14. *Ptosis, cervical sympathetic lesion* A young girl with a right sided ptosis and trophic changes in the fingers. 'Deductive looking' would lead one to suggest that the finger could be due to a burn, gangrene, Raynaud's phenomenon, an embolus, ergotism or a cervical rib. The small pupil with a right sided ptosis were related. The lid of the right side definitely is ptosed since (1) there is overaction on the right, (2) there is a small pupil on the right, (3) the lid cuts tangentially across the small *and* the larger pupil — the right lid must be lower. Relating these two together we have a sympathetic nerve lesion of the eye with the finger change. Diagnosis is a cervical sympathectomy for a severe Raynaud's phenomenon. An alternative possibility is burns in syringomyelia. *(A G M Raynaud, 1834-1881, described 1862.)*
    **psgm**

**15.** a) Atheroma or atherosclerosis
b) Foam cells, cholesterol crystals spaces, recent and previous haemorrhage and increased fibrosis.
cpa

**16.** The hypermobility syndrome, often leading to premature osteoarthrosis.
rh

**17.** a) Single palmar crease (four finger crease, Simian crease); fifth finger clinodactyly.
b) Single palmar crease is present unilaterally in 2 — 4% of the population; fifth finger clinodactyly is present in 0.5 — 1% of the population.
c) Down's syndrome (Trisomy 21)
clge

**18.** Ranula (mucous extravasation cyst).
ofd

**19.** Deformities are characteristic either of cerebral palsy or following a stroke.
clo

**20.** a) Similar vesicles would be found on the feet, shallow ulcers in the mouth and possibly a maculo-papular rash on the buttocks.
b) Yes. It spreads readily within a household.
c) *Coxsackievirus* A16, A10 or A5.
ind

**21.** a) High jugular bulb.
b) No. This may result in severe haemorrhage.
ed

**22.** A ganglion is the commonest tumour arising in the hand. In this case it arose from the inter-carpal joints and was compressing the thenar branch of the median nerve.

If any tumour in the hand is pressing on a vital structure it should be removed.
**Operative Finding:** A ganglion compressing the thenar branch of the median nerve.
hc

**23.** a) A calcified circular cyst in the liver.
b) Hydatid cyst.
c) Suggestive evidence includes the patient's country of origin (Wales, South America, the Middle East, Australia, New Zealand), urticaria or hives. Helpful investigations include eosinophilia, Casoni skin test, complement fixation or other serological test, chest X-ray and a liver scan or CT scan.
d) Aspiration liver biopsy.
e) Surgery may be necessary to remove the intact cyst, or if this is not possible, to marsupialise the cyst and sterilise the contents.
resd

**24.** Hereditary haemorrhagic telangectasia (Rendu — Osler Weber syndrome).
ofd

**25.** This is congenital cataract diagnosed at birth and present with a rubella syndrome.
col

**26.** Body louse.
The body louse *Pediculus humanus* transmits typical epidemic typhus due to *Rickettsia prowazeki,* and Trench Fever. Rickettsial infection is cosmopolitan. The use of DDT for disinfection of louse-infested communities is a primary control measure in epidemic situations.
tmp

27. It is not a stye but an infected meibomian cyst. Treatment however is similar with the application of heat and hot spoon bathings together with an antibiotic ointment.
The patient should be warned that there will be a residual lump within the substance of the lid which will need minor surgery.
**od**

28. The presenting sign is a convergent squint of the left eye. In this case the squint is caused by an opacity within the eye which can be seen as a white area in the pupil. This child was suffering from a retinoblastoma presenting as a large flocculent mass within the globe.
Other conditions presenting like this might be a congenital cataract or inflammation.
The commonest cause of a squint is refractive, i.e. the child needs glasses but this may be complicated by the presence of amblyopia (lazy eye). Thus, all cases of permanent squint should be referred for urgent specialist assessment either to expedite perhaps life-saving therapy in, say, cases of tumour or sight-saving therapy in cases of inflammation.
**od**

29. a) Treacher-Collins syndrome.
b) Deafness.
c) Coloboma of the lower eyelid.
d) 1 in 2.
**clge**

30. An early sign of leprosy, the indeterminate macule, is slightly hypo-pigmented and ill-defined. It retains tactile-sensitivity, sweating function, and hair growth.
**tmp**

31. a) Trophic ulcer.
b) Sensory neuropathy — often associated with peripheral vascular disease.
c) Yes. Insulin is erratically absorbed from lipodystrophic areas. Injection into these areas can, therefore, result in poor control of the diabetes.
**end**

32. *Rickets (vitamin D deficiency)* The classic rosary. The bulges seen on the chest wall at the site of the costo-chondral junctions are produced by the expanded uncalcified matrix. Compare the photograph of the child's wrist, the pathology is the same.
Causes of rickets are: (1) dietary; (2) malabsorption; (3) renal failure; (4) renal tubular defects.
**psgm**

33. Ileocaecal intussusception. A sausage-shaped abdominal mass may be palpable. 90-95 per cent of intussusceptions at this age have no primary cause. In the absence of perforation, shock or advanced intestinal obstruction, hydrostatic reduction with barium enema may be attempted.
**psd**

34. Yes to b). Possibly e).
**bd**

35. Coma in malignant tertian malaria due to *Plasmodium falciparum*. This is one of the commonest and most lethal complications.
Confusion is an early warning sign.
**tmp**

36. *Schistosomiasis.*
Haematuria, often at the end of urination, is a characteristic early clinical feature of infection with this parasite. Typical terminal spined eggs of *S. haematobium* may be found in the centrifuge deposit.
**tmp**

37. *Galactorrhoea* An acromegalic with hyperprolactinaemia: Milking of the breast and squeezing of the nipple increases the flow. Galactorrhoea may be caused by: (1) drugs — phenothiazines, oral contraceptives, reserpine, tricyclic antidepressants; (2) pituitary tumours; (3) hypothalmic disease; (4) 'ectopic' prolactin production — lung tumours; (5) primary hypothyroidism; (6) chest wall injury — trauma, surgery, herpes zoster, by afferent reflex stimulation.
The mammary tissue develops under the influence of oestrogens — this produces the pubescent breast. Circulating prolactin induces nipple and areolar development and later secretion.
**psgm**

38. Ankylosing spondylitis and Reiter's syndrome.
**rh**

39. Larvae of the Tumbu fly *(Cordylobia anthropophaga)*. Multiple infections cause painful boils on the skin of the trunk or limbs.
**tmp**

40. A Heberden's node due to osteoarthrosis.
**rh**

41. *Hypertrophic pulmonary osteo-arthropathy* Swelling of the terminal phalanx of the fingers is present but there is marked curvature of the nail with loss of the normal obtuse angle at the nail fold. This is gross clubbing. The patient complained of pain in the joints of the extremities. On the X-ray periosteal bone reaction can be seen on the metacarpal of the thumb *(arrow)*. Periosteal reaction is much more common on the bones of the forearms and legs. This patient had bronchiectasis but by far the commonest cause is a carcinoma of the bronchus.
**psgm**

42. Appearances are exactly similar in both tuberculosis and rheumatoid arthritis. Aspiration and radiography will establish the diagnosis.
**clo**

43. Psoriatic arthritis — typical nail dystrophy with inflammatory arthritis of the terminal interphalangeal joints.
**rh**

44. Hypospadias.
Caused by failure of closure of the urethral groove as a consequence of which the urethral opening lies on the ventral aspect of the penis. The anomaly is classified according to the site of opening of the urethra — glandular, penile, penoscrotal and perineal. The redundant foreskin on the dorsal aspect of the penis characteristically forms a 'hood'. This is a constant feature of all hypospadias. The redundant foreskin is used in the repair of the anomaly. Circumcision is absolutely contraindicated in the presence of hypospadias. The parents frequently complain that the child is unable to micturate while standing without wetting his trousers or shoes. Treatment is best carried out during the 3rd or 4th year of life.
**psd**

45. The distended abdomen and visible peristalsis. The baby has low intestinal obstruction. X-ray examination in upright position after some fluid intake will show multiple fluid levels.
**pd**

46. Allergic manifestation to eye drops, particularly some antibiotics and miotics used in the therapy of glaucoma.
Here the acute eczematous changes include the upper and lower eyelid, but if the condition is chronic and involves only the upper eyelids cosmetics should be suspected.
od

47. *Psoriatic arthropathy* The full blown picture. The terminal IP joint swelling can be seen in the little and ring fingers. There is nail ridging, the pitting is visible in the close up and the plaque of psoriasis is seen in the bottom left hand corner on the wrist.
psgm

48. Chagas' disease caused by *Trypanosoma cruzi*. Mural thrombi may be present at the apex of the left ventricle, with marked thinning of both ventricular walls. Apical aneurysmal formation is commonly seen.
tmp

49. Proteinuria and/or nephrotic syndrome.
rd

50. b) Psoriasis.
bd

51. Untreated torticollis (wry neck).
clo

52. Diabetes mellitus.
rd

53. c) Pulmonary fat embolism.
chtr

54. Dental cyst.
ofd

55. Nephroblastoma (Wilms' tumour). Most common intra-renal malignant tumour of childhood. Peak age of incidence is three to four years. Presenting symptom is most frequently an increase in the size of the abdomen or an abdominal mass found incidentally during bathing or on routine physical examination. The mass is firm and smooth and arises out of the flank, but may cross the midline. The prognosis for Wilms' tumour is generally excellent in contrast to the poor outlook for the child with neuroblastoma which is usually widely disseminated at the time of diagnosis.
psd

56. Adult polycystic disease; renal failure in middle age hypertension.
rd

57. Hydrops cornea due to Descemet's Rupture, commonly seen in advanced keratoconus and eye rubbing.
col

58. *Jaundice* The shininess of the nail due to the polishing effect of using the fingers to scratch the back which itched. Patient was a 42-year-old man with a stone in a common bile duct.
Note the *polished nail tip* is caused by scratching the skin. Cosmetic polishing makes the whole nail shine. Pruritus may be due to: (1) parasitic infestations: scabies, pediculosis; (2) eczema; (3) liver disease (even preceding jaundice); (4) drug reactions; (5) malignant disease (lymphoma, leukaemia, carcinoma); (6) metabolic disease (diabetes mellitus, uraemia); (7) old age.
psgm

59. A nail fold lesion due to vasculitis most commonly seen in rheumatoid arthritis.
rh

60. Migrating larvae of *S. stercoralis* in skin. Auto-infection can lead to severe 'creeping eruption' usually in the back. This may occur many years (30 or more) after initial infection. Deep migration of the larvae may be associated with 'eosinophilic lung' type of syndrome.
tmp

61. Papillary necrosis; diabetes mellitus, analgesic abuse.
rd

62. Renal calculi; medullary sponge kidney.
rd

63. a) X-linked mental retardation with macro-orchidism (large testes).
    b) Chromosome analysis specifying that one was looking for a "Fragile-X" chromosome. The cells would then be cultured in folate free medium to demonstrate the characteristic fragile site at the distal end of the long arm of the X-chromosome.
clge

64. *Ampicillin; infectious mononucleosis* — beware pharyngitis with small ulcers; take a throat swab and/or prescribe a different antibiotic.
psgm

65. Chronic tophaceous gout.
rh

66. Partial precocious puberty is mostly benign and maturation proceeds normally. The size of the breasts may differ.
pd

67. *Ainhum* Aetiology unknown. Common in West Africa amongst those who go barefoot. An initial constriction at the base of the little toe tightens like a tourniquet and ultimately the toe falls off or is knocked off. Treatment is to amputate — the next toe may be involved. The pathology is just fibrous tissue at the base of the toe. There is no neurological or vascular defect nor systemic illness.
psgm

68. Xanthogranulomatous pyelonephritis.
rd

69. (1) pars flaccida; (2) pars tensa; (3) short process of the malleus; (4) long process of the malleus; (5) light reflection; (6) vascular strip; (7) recess for the round window; (8) recess for the eustachian tube.
ed

70. Rheumatoid arthritis.
rh

71. The risks of injecting tendon with steroid. This is partial rupture of the Achilles tendon in a patient who has had an injection of Hydrocortisone into the tendon.
is

72. Main d'accoucher; Ca and/or Mg deficiency.
nd

73. a) Septic flexor tenosynovitis of the right middle finger.
    b) Early incision and drainage of the flexor tendon sheath to avoid necrosis and rupture of the flexor tendons.
hc

74. a) Neoplasm of the external auditory canal.

b) Biopsy. Pathological examination revealed an adenocarcinoma.
**ed**

75. An interdigital neuroma being removed at operation. The condition is known as Morton's metatarsalgia and the symptoms are pain between the metatarsal heads on weight-bearing. Not an uncommon condition among runners.
**is**

76. Squamous cell carcinoma.
**ofd**

77. Idiopathic retroperitoneal fibrosis (RPF).
**ur**

78. c) and e).
**gem**

79. Peutz-Jegher's disease.
**ofd**

80. Facioscapulohumeral dystrophy (Dejerine myopathy).
**clo**

81. The baby on the left is hypothyroid; the "normal" looking one in the middle is a mosaic and the one on the right has Down's syndrome.
**pd**

82. a), b), c) and d).
**nb**

83. Cigarette burn. Child abuse. The diagnosis of child abuse should be considered carefully when there is an apparent discrepancy between the time of injury and attendance at the consulting rooms; or where there are other signs of abuse, such as bruises, unexplained fractures, 'pulled elbow', malnutrition.
**psd**

84. b) and c).
**bd**

85. *Prayer callus* The Moslem priest prays assiduously several times a day, prayer involving the forehead touching the ground. This man — one of a group visiting this country, in common with his colleagues, had a callosity on his forehead from many years of prayer (*arrowed*).
**psgm**

86. Myelomatosis.
**rd**

87. a) No. The white exudate strictly confined to the tonsils is very characteristic of infectious mononucleosis.
b) Generalised enlargement of lymph nodes and splenomegaly would be helpful in supporting the diagnosis.
c) A white blood cell count and a heterophile antibody test, such as the Paul Bunnell test or Monospot test.
**ind**

88. a) Primary acquired cholesteatoma.
b) Bone resorption in the area of the pars flaccida by the enlarging cholesteatoma.
**ed**

89. Loss of sensation, ischaemia and sepsis all contribute to this lesion.
**di**

90. Acute dental abscess upper first molar.
**ofd**

91. *Sickle cell anaemia* Dactylitis in a small child with bone infarction producing an acute, tender swelling of the finger. Differential diagnosis between sepsis, acute or chronic

(tuberculosis), syphilis, sickle cell disease, sarcoidosis.

**psgm**

**92.** a) Yes. b) Yes. c) No, but he may have a cough. d) Typhoid or paratyphoid fever.

**ind**

**93.** Anal fissure. Most common cause of rectal bleeding in first year of life. Usually located in the midline of the anus — anterior or posteriorly. Develops after the passage of a large constipated stool. Treatment consists of mild laxatives to produce a softish but formed stool, local analgesic ointments to relieve the pain and regular digital anal dilatation until the fissures are completely healed (7-10 days). Untreated the condition may lead to a secondary megacolon due to prolonged voluntary retention of stool.

**psd**

**94.** a) Serous otitis media, right ear.
b) Approximately 25 dB.
c) Mechanical obstruction of the eustachian tube or past history of otitis media.

**ed**

**95.** Torus platinus.

**ofd**

**96.** Footballer's ankle, i.e. marginal impingement exostoses around the ankle.
It is not degenerative joint disease (osteoarthrosis) since there is no narrowing of the joint gap.

**is**

**97.** Bitot's spot; no.

**nd**

**98.** a) Primary herpetic gingivostomatitis.
b) *Herpesvirus hominis* type 1.

c) About 60%.

**ind**

**99.** a) Acute conjunctivitis. Treatment is vigorous and usually means application of a suitable antibiotic drop like Chloramphenicol, with antibiotic ointment at night.
b) Should the case not respond in seven to ten days the diagnosis should be reconsidered.
NEVER make a diagnosis of monocular conjunctivitis as it pre-supposes that a monocular conjunctivitis is not infective, i.e. it must be secondary to other pathology: that is a missed foreign body, blocked tear passages or what is more likely it may not be a conjunctivitis at all but perhaps an acute iridocyclitis, acute glaucoma or a corneal ulcer.

**od**

**100.** Chronic pyelonephritis.

**rd**

**101.** Erythema nodosum.

**rh**

**102.** *Caroteneaemia* Yellow pigmentation due to carotene. This is caused by (1) excess carotene intake — overeating mangoes, carrots (4kg a day!), pawpaw, oranges; (2) myxoedema — high levels of carotene due to a defect of enzymatic conversion to vitamin A; (3) an association with hyperbetalipoproteinaemia.

**psgm**

**103.** a) Yes. There is usually severe ulceration of the buccal mucosa and inflammation of the conjunctivae and external genitalia.
b) Toxic epidermal necrolysis or scalded-skin syndrome.

256

c) This may be caused by *Staphylococcus aureus* infection or may be drug-induced.
**ind**

**104.** He suffers from the *tarda* form of osteogenesis imperfecta (brittle bones). The congenital form of this disease is apparent at birth with multiple fractures, the tarda form develops later and there may be a history of one or more fractures.
**clo**

**105.** Tennis elbow or lateral epicondylitis treated by steroid injection. Note site of loss of pigmentation and thinning of skin (steroid stigmata) over lateral epicondyle.
**is**

**106.** a) Myotonic dystrophy.
b) 1 in 2.
c) Clinical examination plus EMG plus slit lamp examination to look for lens opacities.
d) Yes — in some families. The myotonic dystrophy gene is linked to the ABH secretor gene. However, not all families are informative.
**clge**

**107.** *Holmes-Adie syndrome, the myotonic pupil* In the dark the pupils are equal and dilated. In sunlight the left pupil has constricted much more quickly than the right which comes down very slowly and once contracted will dilate again only slowly — the tonic pupil. It may be associated.with absence of the tendon reflexes and is a benign condition which is important as a differential diagnosis from tabes dorsalis. (The difficulty in reading may be due to slowness in accommodation).
**psgm**

**108.** Tubular carcinoma.
**rd**

**109.** By establishing the diagnosis; by influencing clinical treatment and management.
**rd**

**110.** *Gouty tophus* The deposition of uric acid in the cartilage of the ear may be seen as small, white excresences on the helix. They may be confused with Darwin's tubercle and should be looked for diligently.
This one is easily seen and should be contrasted with the less prominent Darwin's tubercle (*arrowed*) of the ear.
**psgm**

**111.** Fat Embolism.
**chtr**

**112.** a) There are dilated retinal veins, multiple retinal haemorrhages and a swollen, congested optic disc; they are caused by central retinal vein occlusion.
b) Hypertension, hyperlipidaemia, hyperviscosity of the blood, diabetes mellitus.
**esd**

**113.** 'Salivary' adenoma or adenocarcinoma.
**ofd**

**114.** 'Flag' sign or signa de bandera.
**nd**

**115.** Left incomplete indirect inguinal hernia in a male infant. The bulge in the groin does not extend down into the scrotum. This type of hernia is commonly seen by the parents or family practitioner and frequently cannot be demonstrated during consultation. In infants under six months of age, surgery should be performed as soon as convenient as there is a high incidence of irreducibility. After six months of age the procedure is no longer a matter of urgency.

**psd**

116. a) Ask exactly what the patient was doing. If he says
    (a) I was using a hammer and chisel on concrete
    or (b) using a grinding wheel without protective goggles
    refer the case immediately, as in these occupational hazards the patient may have sustained an injury as evidenced in the photograph by an iris prolapse and a distorted pupil.
    b) Penetrating eye injury with prolapsed intra-ocular contents. Refer the patient immediately. Do not apply any tight dressings as more intra-ocular contents may be expelled. Keep the intra-ocular pressure as even as possible and refer immediately.

**od**

117. Pellagra.

**nd**

118. b) Ecchymotic mask.

**chtr**

119. d) Hiatus Hernia.

**ent**

120. Xerophthalmia due to vitamin A deficiency.

**nd**

121. a) Deep (thenar) space infection.
    b) Suppuration (because of the persisting throbbing pain).
    c) Incision and drainage. Decompress the carpal tunnel. Beware of the median nerve and its thenar branch.

**hc**

122. a) Dental.

**ent**

123. a) Familial shortness of stature; major systemic illness; social deprivation (illustrated). Endocrine, chromosomal and developmental causes of growth retardation are uncommon.
    b) Bone age is increased in adrenocortical overactivity and reduced in growth hormone deficiency.

**end**

124. Phimosis. The preputial orifice is narrowed and scarred by fibrous tissue. Usually follows repeated attempts at retraction by medical attendant or parents. The trauma causes splitting of the foreskin and subsequent healing occurs by fibrosis. Rare in boys under 5 to 6 years of age. Definite indication for circumcision. Contraindications to circumcision are hypospadias and ammoniacal dermititis (nappy rash). In hypospadias the hooded foreskin is required for the surgical correction and ammoniacal dermatitis may lead to meatal ulceration of the unprotected glans

**psd**

125. a) This is geographic tongue (erythema migrans) in which loss of filiform papillae occurs temporarily. The lesions appear to move over the surface of the tongue because of their rapid appearance and disappearance.
    b) There is no known associated generalised precipitating factor.
    c) There is no known treatment. Reassurance is very important as the patients often suspect malignancy.

**om**

126. High speed falls when water-skiing may lead to forced douches of the

vagina causing peritonitis in female water-skiers who do not wear suitable protective clothing.
**is**

127. d) Tophaceous gout.
**gem**

128. The condition is a CAVERNOUS SINUS THROMBOSIS which despite antibiotics has a high mortality rate. Squeezing of boils, especially in the area of the face, is thought to be dangerous due to spreading the infection via the veins.
**gsd**

129. Fluorosis.
**nd**

130. The child suffers from congenital absence of muscle development around all joints which were stiff and contracted. The condition is known as arthrogryposis multiplex congenita. In the commonest type the lower limbs only are affected.
**clo**

131. Oxy(acro)cephaly due to early closure of the coronal sutures appears with other abnormalities of face and orbit. Increasing intracranial pressure leads to visual and cerebral damage.
**pd**

132. The patient had acute osteomyelitis in childhood, leading to destruction of the upper tibial growth-plate.
**clo**

133. Perlèche.
**nd**

134. Nutritional rickets due to inadequate Vitamin D intake. The swelling is due to enlargement of the lower ends of the radius and ulna, where most growth occurs.
**clo**

135. Ocular complications of a 'black eye' are easily diagnosed with the aid of a hand torch and ophthalmoscope.
The use of a hand torch may show the presence of blood in the anterior chamber or rupture of the globe.
The use of the ophthalmoscope may show the presence of retinal changes.
Any orbital complications may be diagnosed by the subjective signs of diplipia or the demonstration of limited eye movements.
**od**

136. a) Splinter haemorrhages.
b) Subacute bacterial endocarditis.
**ind**

137. Jaundice, neck retraction, extensor spasm of the limbs with clenched fists due to kernicterus, the neurotoxic effect of hyperbilirubinaemia (serum level in excess of 20mg/dl). Severe motor and intellectual disability results.
**pd**

138. Gouty tophus.
**clo**

139. Contracture of tenso fascia femoris muscle following poliomyelitis. Because the muscle traverses both hip and knee joints it can produce flexion deformity at both joints simultaneously.
**clo**

140. Complete rupture of long head of biceps. No specific treatment required other than exercise to restore normal function in the arm.
**is**

**141.** a) Blue sclerae and opalescent teeth (dentinogenesis imperfecta).
b) Osteogenesis imperfecta.
clge

**142.** Umbilical granuloma. An umbilical granuloma is simply an overgrowth of granulation tissue at the site of attachment of the normal umbilical cord. Produces a bloodstained discharge. The condition must be differentiated from a remnant of the omphalomesenteric duct which may have a patent communication with the small intestine. Responds to cauterisation with silver nitrate or to simple ligation of the stalk at its base.
psd

**143.** a) This is a characteristic picture of phenytoin (epanutin) induced hyperplasia.
b) Widespread hyperplastic gingivitis may occur during pregnancy.
c) Strict oral hygiene measures reduce the exaggerated inflammatory response both in phenytoin-induced and in-pregnancy-gingivitis.
om

**144.** Thyroglossal cyst. May form anywhere along the pathway of the persisting thyroglossal tract which extends from the foramen caecum of the tongue to the pyramidal lobe of the thyroid gland. More commonly located at the level of the hyoid bone and presents as an asymptomatic lump in the midline of the neck. Treatment consists of excision of the entire thyroglossal tract including the central portion of the hyoid bone. The child should be referred for surgery before the cyst becomes infected. The recurrence rate after previous infection is high.

Early surgical excision is therefore recommended.
psd

**145.** a) This is carcinoma of the lip.
b) This is much more common in elderly males and is characteristically painless and slow growing.
c) It is often mistaken for a long-standing lesion of herpes.
om

**146.** a) The site is unusual for erysipelas but common for anthrax. Moreover, severe oedema is a prominent feature of anthrax.
b) Blood cultures may be positive in severe anthrax.
ind

**147.** Pes calcaneo-cavus following poliomyelitis. The deformity is due to imbalance between relatively strong extensor muscles of ankle and foot and a paralysed calf muscle.
clo

**148.** b) Round window.
ent

**149.** a) Hypertrophy of the interventricular septum disproportionate to the left ventricular free wall.
b) Primary cardiomyopathy, hypertrophic type with an asymmetrical pattern.
cpa

**150.** a) Tympanosclerosis.
b) Prior otitis media.
ed

**151.** Bilateral pes cavus. It can be due to a variety of diseases — either an inherited neurological disorder, or associated with spinal dysraphism, or spina bifida.
clo

**152.** Rheumatoid arthritis can lead to spontaneous rupture of tendons.
clo

**153.** a) The patient is female, probably pregnant since striae gravidarum are present and look recent. The impression left by a fetal stethoscope also suggests pregnancy with oedema of the abdominal wall present.
b) The presence of abdominal oedema suggesting that the patient may have excessive weight gain and possibly pre-eclampsia.
clgy

**154.** Undescended testis. The finger is referring to the position of the right testis in the superficial inguinal pouch. For fertility reasons treatment is optimally undertaken during the second year of life. Delayed treatment exposes the child to the risk of sterility, trauma or torsion of the undescended testis. The long-term risk is that of malignancy — teratoma or seminoma (40x greater than the average population). Orchidopexy does not reduce the risk of malignancy, it merely facilitates early diagnosis.
psd

**155.** a) de Quervain's frictional tenosynovitis, osteoarthritis of the carpo-metacarpal joint of the thumb. Fracture of the scaphoid, ganglion cyst of the wrist joint.
b) Rest the wrist on a splint. Cortico-steroid injection. Operative decompression if conservative measures fail.
hc

**156.** a) This is a characteristic Aspirin burn. Such a lesion can be produced by dissolving a single tablet containing aspirin in the area.
b) The origin of the pain is usually evident, as in this case, from a nearby carious or heavily filled tooth.
c) The burn maybe treated by mild antiseptics but the definitive treatment is of the dental condition.
om

**157.** d). Neglect
gem

**158.** a) Pernicious anaemia.
b) This is not a specific pattern. A very similar picture may occur in folate deficiency or iron deficiency.
c) The glossitis may occur very early in the onset of pernicious anaemia, before the erythrocytes are affected. A simple blood count might, therefore, not be of help in diagnosis without a full screen.
om

**159.** The "sign of the setting sun", a transitory phenomenon in newborn and prematures with birth shock. Persistency points to severe brain damage.
pd

**160.** This is a dry eye problem — early Sjögrens Syndrome.
col

**161.** "Tramline" calcifications in this case of encephalotrigeminal angiomatosis (Sturge-Weber-Dimitri syndrome). Ocular and cerebral damage will develop.
pd

**162.** a) Scarlet fever.
b) The fur would peel leaving a red-strawberry tongue.
ind

**163.** a) Pregnancy, Ovarian cyst, enlarged uterus with fibroid(s).

b) Ensure that the bladder was empty if necessary by passing a catheter.

**clgy**

**164.** Epididymitis is rare at this age. Torsion of testis should be suspected and the area explored urgently to prevent gangrene. A bilateral condition may be associated with mumps.

**gsd**

**165.** Tuberculosis of the right sacro-iliac joint with a 'cold' abscess.

**clo**

**166.** a) Heberden's node, rheumatoid nodule, ganglion cyst, giant cell tumour of tendon sheath. Primary or secondary bone tumour.

b) An X-ray shows secondary bone erosion at the head of the middle phalanx.

c) Adequate exposure and removal after protecting vital deep structures of the neurovascular bundles tendon and joint mechanism.

**hc**

**167.** Syringomyelia resulting in destructive arthropathy of the shoulder joint (Charcot joint).

**clo**

**168.** Psoriatic arthropathy.

**clo**

**169.** Trichomonas vaginitis. The protozoa is partly anaerobic hence the small bubbles produced. Oral Metronidazole is the recommended treatment.

**clgy**

**170.** Multiple fractures (Osteogenesis imperfecta).

**ofd**

**171.** 'Monkey' Facies; marasmus.

**nd**

**172.** Foetus-to-foetus transfusion (intra-uterine transfusion syndrome) via an arterio-venous shunt. The donor is anaemic and dystrophic, the recipient has severe plethora.

**pd**

**173.** b) Ludvig's angina.

**ent**

**174.** a) Pulp space infection, osteomyelitis, granuloma (rheumatoid), neoplasm.

b) An X-ray showed a punched-out area of distal phalanx.

c) Biopsy. This showed secondary carcinoma. The primary was in the lung.

**hc**

**175.** a) Infection — soft tissue infection, deep tendon, bone of joint infection. Inflammatory and metabolic conditions — gout, rheumatoid synovitis, etc., acute calcification.

b) Investigations — full blood count, serum uric acid (this was raised). Aspirate and analyse the fluid obtained. Arrange rheumatoid tests, e.g. Latex if suspect rheumatoid arthritis.

c) Anti-gout treatment. Incise and drain if suspect an infective process.

**hc**

**176.** The patient suffers from haemophilia. This is a sex-linked disorder affecting males only and transmitted by the female. The symptoms are due to impairment of clotting factors in the blood. It can lead to severe derangement of joints

due to repeated inter-articular haemorrhage.
clo

177.  a) Lip swelling may occur in oral Crohn's disease.
      b) Angular cheilitis, cervical lymph node enlargement and fissuring and tuberculoid granulomas may occur in the mouth.
      c) The important long term factor is to observe for the possible onset of lesions in other part of the gastrointestinal tract. The incidence of this in these patients is not yet known.
      om

178.  Advanced giant cell tumour of the lower end of the radius.
      clo

179.  a), b) and c).
      gem

180.  a) Infected subtotal perforation of the right tympanic membrane.
      b) *Pseudomonas* or *staphylococcus.*
      c) Topical antibiotics are most effective.
      ed

181.  Lipoatrophy at abdominal injection sites of insulin in adolescent diabetic.
      di

182.  He is suffering from ankylosing spondylitis. Diagnosis is confirmed by a high sedimentation rate and a radiograph of the sacro-iliac joints which are obliterated early in this disease.
      clo

183.  This is necrobiosis lipoidica occurring in diabetes.
      di

184.  a) Primary infection with *Herpesvirus hominis,* usually type 1.
      b) Yes. Doctors and nurses are at risk from patients.
      ind

185.  Sixth nerve palsy and seventh nerve palsy, both on the right, occurring in diabetes.
      di

186.  a) Well-demarcated cannonball shadows throughout both lungs.
      b) Metastases from a carcinoma of colon, stomach, thyroid, bronchus, prostate, kidney or breast. The differential diagnosis includes tuberculosis, sarcoidosis, reticulosis, rheumatoid lung, Wegener's granulomatosis or staphylococcal septicaemia.
      c) It depends upon other physical signs which may suggest the site of the primary tumour. Direct biopsy of the lung is the most fruitful, and aspiration liver biopsy is also helpful. Sputum examination would be of value if due to tuberculosis or staphylococcal pneumonia.
      d) Metastatic carcinoma of the prostate by oestrogens and castration, breast by oophorectomy and tamoxifen, bronchus by combined chemotherapy. There is no worthwhile treatment of metastases from alimentary tract cancer.
      resd

187.  The mother had poorly controlled diabetes.
      di

188.  c) Suspicious of a tonsillar neoplasm.
      ent

**189.** a) Bilateral solid breast shadows.

b) Bilateral opaque silicone-filled prosthetic implants for cosmetic enlargement of the breasts.

c) They do not cause diagnostic confusion (once seen never forgotten) but they may obscure lesions in the underlying lung. Beware of air-containing balloon implants. Obeying laws of physics, they enlarge when a patient is airborne and may become very tense and uncomfortable.

resd

**190.** a) This is a typical minor aphthous ulcer.

b) The important differential diagnosis in all oral ulceration is from carcinoma.

c) In about 5% of adult patients aphthous ulceration is associated with hitherto unsuspected asymptomatic Coeliac disease.

om

**191.** Dermatitis seborrhoides (Moro), appears within the first trimester, more frequently in breast-fed infants. The distribution of the rash differs from that of infantile eczema. There is usually no recurrence after treatment.

pd

**192.** a) Lichen planus. This is the reticular non-erosive form.

b) Painful erosive lesions may occur.

c) Treatment of the erosive lesions is with local steroids, antibiotics, and antiseptics. The non-erosive lesions are resistant to treatment.

om

**193.** Oil cancer of scrotum.

ur

**194.** a) Round window niche.

b) Perforations of this sort usually heal spontaneously.

ed

**195.** b) Gerontoxon.

gem

**196.** a) The very dense enlarged right clavicle is the clue to the diagnosis of Paget's disease, which causes high-output cardiac failure.

b) No, not necessary in this instance.

c) The pleural transudate is due to cardiac failure.

d) There will be other physical signs of high output cardiac failure and of Paget's disease. X-rays of other bones will show characteristic changes of Paget's disease. The skull X-ray shows a fluffy cotton-wool appearance. There is increased resorption together with increased bone formation. Biochemical changes comprise raised serum alkaline phosphatase level and increased hydroxyprolinuria.

e) Sir James Paget (1814-1899) was surgeon to Queen Victoria and to St. Bartholomew's Hospital, London; President of the Royal College of Surgeons; Vice-Chancellor of the University of London.

f) Cardiac failure, fractures, compressive neurological syndromes, deafness, osteosarcoma.

g) Treatments include simple analgesics, calcitonin, mithramycin, diphosphonates.

resd

**197.** a) This is a case of a ganglion cyst arising from the distal inter-phalangeal joint pressing on the root of the nail, causing the

ridging. Recurrent breaking down of this cyst produces the discharge of synovial fluid.
b) Resect the cyst and the underlying bone spur at the distal inter-phalangeal joint. Injection of cortico-steroid is sometimes advocated, but such treatment can lead to atrophy and infection.

hc

**198.** Congenital arterio-venous aneurysm.

clo

**199.** A rare metabolic disorder known as Alkaptonuria (ochronosis).

clo

**200.** a) Acute external otitis.
b) *Staphylococcus aureus* and *pseudomonas aeuruginosa.*

ed

**201.** a) A thin wisp of barium is seen within a normal appendix. A thin white line of barium is also seen within an intestinal helminth giving the appearance of a barium meal within a barium meal. A flocculation pattern of barium is also evident.
b) Roundworm infestation (ascariasis).
c) Ascaris lumbricoides is found in faeces. There is accompanying eosinophilia and elevated serum IgE levels.
d) Piperazine 10 Gram in a single dose, repeated after 2 or 3 weeks.

resd

**202.** a), b), c) and e).

dy

**203.** A simple ganglion arising from the ankle joint.

clo

**204.** b) and c).

ld

**205.** a) Thyroid nodule.
b) Serum thyroxine (and triiodothyronine); thyroid scan.

end

**206.** d) Further investigation.

ent

**207.** Bilateral cataracts due to poorly controlled diabetes.

di

**208.** a) Dysphasia — an inability to exchange spoken or written ideas normally when the mechanisms of speech and writing are intact and the patient is not demented, blind or deaf.
b) It implies the presence of a cortical lesion which will be in the left hemisphere of those who are naturally right-handed, and of some who are left-handed. A non-fluent dysphasia of this sort, in which the patient is clearly aware of his disability, is caused by a lesion involving Broca's area around the lower part of the precentral gyrus.
c) Cerebrovascular accidents and tumours.

cln

**209.** b) and c).

ld

**210.** a) A myxoma of the heart.
b) The inter-atrial septal wall of the left atrium.
c) A myxoma consists of weakly eosinophilic and basophilic matrix containing scattered stellate and lipidic cells, fibrocytes, occasional blood vessels and scanty haemorrhage with the surface covered by endothelium.

cpa

**211.** a) Chronic paronychia, squamous cell carcinoma of the nail bed.
b) Remove the nail and biopsy the nail bed. This showed squamous cell carcinoma. This patient required treatment for the squamous cell carcinoma of his thumb, and for the metastatic lymph nodes in the axilla.
N.B.: Any chronic lesion should be biopsied.
hc

**212.** Cancer of the male breast does occur and unfortunately tends to spread rapidly with fixity of the tumour to muscle and skin and extension to lymph glands.
gsd

**213.** a) Senile calcific aortic valve stenosis.
b) This is a tricuspid aortic valve with nodular calcified masses on the aortic side of cusps. There are no adhesions of the commissures and the free edges are not involved.
cpa

**214.** b), c), d) and e).
ld

**215.** Rheumatoid polyarthritis in the hands, usually starts at the metacarpophalangeal joints.
clo

**216.** d) A foreign body.
ent

**217.** a) Bullous myringitis.
b) *Mycoplasma pneumoniae*.
ed

**218.** Marginal Ulceration, possibly Moorens type — unknown aetiology.
col

**219.** b) A right tension pneumothorax.
chtr

**220.** Bilateral rheumatoid arthritis, which is the only common cause of bilateral gleno-humeral disease.
clo

**221.** a), b) and e).
ld

**222.** a), b), d) and e).
dy

**223.** c) Swimming.
ent

**224.** d) Lichen simplex.
dy

**225.** a) Lesch-Nyhan disease.
b) Raised uric acid and absenthypoxanthine-gusnine-phosphoribosyl transferase (HGPRT).
c) Yes — by doing the appropriate enzyme test on cells grown from the amniotic fluid.
clge

**226.** The cornea will eventually become chronically oedematous, uveitis and cataract develop and permanent blindness is likely.
col

**227.** b) A chylothorax when opening the pleural cavity.
chtr

**228.** Horseshoe kidney. Medially facing calyx on left.
ur

**229.** b) Staphlococcus aureus.
dy

**230.** e) Psoriasis.
dy

**231.** Osteochondritis of the capitellum in a child (epiphyseal lines clearly shown). An overuse injury in a young gymnast leading to loose body formation and severe damage to the elbow joint. An example of unacceptable overuse injury in sport in children.
is

**232.** d) Aphthous.
ent

**233.** Chronic trauma from wearing hard corneal contact lenses, response is called Follicular Palpebral Conjunctivitis.
col

**234.** b) Bowen's Disease
To exclude the possibility of infiltrating squamous cell carcinoma arising in the lesion.
sp

**235.** Phenylpyruvic acid and metabolites above normal concentration. A case of phenylketonuria.
pd

**236.** The Ehlos-Dandros syndrome in which there is excessive mobility of joints varying from mild ligamentous laxity to a more severe widespread disorder; rarely severe cardio-vascular abnormalities develop in later life.
clo

**237.** c) Tumoural calcinosis.
bd

**238.** c) and e).
dy

**239.** a), b), d) and e).
gem

**240.** a) Any open wound to a finger may have divided all structures beneath that wound. In this case there was division of the flexor profundus, partial division of the flexor superficialis, partial division of the radial border digital nerve, and division of the radial border digital artery.
b) Referral to a specialist for repair of the divided structures. (Doctors without experience in hand surgery should not attempt the repair of such vital structures as nerves and tendons in the hand, because the complication rate of inexpert repairs is very high, most patients developing severe stiffness and other complications). Ideally, such referral and repair should be within 24 to 48 hours after injury.
hc

**241.** Hypopyon Ulceration. In this patient due to Pyocyoneus infection from soft lens wear (with a dry eye problem).
col

**242.** a) Apert's syndrome.
b) Syndactyly of fingers and toes; craniostenosis, narrow or cleft palate, mental retardation.
c) This is an autosomal dominant condition, if parents are normal then the affected child must have arisen as a new mutation. Recurrence risks would be very small.
clge

**243.** Cannonball secondaries, frequently produced by carcinoma of kidney.
ur

**244.** b) and d).
dy

**245.** Cullen. It is a sign of intraperitoneal bleeding. In this case, due to an

ectopic pregnancy.
clgy

**246.** c) The chorda tympani.
ent

**247.** Carcinoma left kidney with classical pathological circulation.
ur

**248.** a) Sturge-Weber syndrome.
b) Not genetic and therefore very small.
c) Left side.
d) Tram-line calcification.
e) Buphthalmos.
clge

**249.** The patient suffers from multiple neurofibromatosis. Presentation varies from a single innocent tumour as shown in the photograph to a widespread condition affecting virtually the whole body and it can be associated with severe scoliosis.
clo

**250.** a), c), d) and e).
ld

**251.** a) Ophthalmopathy associated with Graves' disease.
b) Serum thyroxine; thyroid antibodies.
c) Upper lid retraction; proptosis; periorbital oedema; conjunctival injection.
end

**252.** Paget's disease of bone.
clo

**253.** d) and e).
dy

**254.** Obviously carcinoma has to be considered apart from any of the usual lesions which may be noted in a hair-bearing area of skin. This is, in fact, an hidradena (sweatgland tumour) of the vulva which can

mimic a carcinoma.
clgy

**255.** This is characteristic of vibration tool disease where digital arterial spasm and blockage result from the vibration of power tools, e.g. grinding and pneumatic tools and mechanical chisels.
pvd

**256.** b) and d).
dy

**257.** Splinter haemorrhages in the nail folds indicate an underlying vasculitis associated with disseminated lupus erythematosus, rheumatoid arthritis and polyarteritis nodosa.
pvd

**258.** Secondary deposit in the terminal phalanx from a carcinoma of the rectum.
clo

**259.** A slowly growing solid tumour in this area is most likely to be a mixed tumour of the parotid. An adenolymphoma is softer, a sebaceous cyst or lymphatic gland more superficial and a CAROTID body tumour of this size is usually a little lower.
gsd

**260.** c) and d).
gem

**261.** a) Crush injury of the chest.
chtr

**262.** a) This is a case of high pressure injection injury. The combined effect of high pressure and toxaemia in the closed tissue space of the distal pulp produces cellulitis, vasculitis, thrombosis, and reactive fibrosis.
b) This is an emergency, and within

hours radical incision and debridement should be carried out to prevent spreading necrosis leading to gangrene of the digits.
**hc**

**263.** a), c) and e).
**ld**

**264.** The first manifestation of rheumatoid polyarthritis can be a local chronic bursal enlargement.
**clo**

**265.** Typical of phlegmasia caerulea dolens. Pressure must be relieved by thrombectomy, followed by heparin.
**pvd**

**266.** Temporal arteritis which is not uncommon and is confirmed by biopsy.
**pvd**

**267.** c) When there is fresh bleeding.
**ent**

**268.** Jaundice and a glass eye was usually associated with a previous melanoma of an eye followed later by spread to the liver. In this case it was not so — she had a cancer of the pancreas.
**gsd**

**269.** b), c), d) and e).
**dy**

**270.** b), c) and e).
**ld**

**271.** a) Heterochromia
b) Waardenburg
c) Deafness
d) No — only about 20%
e) 1 in 2
**clge**

**272.** c) Infectious mononeucleosis.
**ent**

**273.** **Left** — both kidneys functioning, non invasive papillary neoplasm.
**Right** — non functioning left kidney, solid invasive neoplasm.
**ur**

**274.** a) Cushing's syndrome.
b) Steroid drug therapy is the commonest cause in both sexes. The commonest cause in males not taking steroids is the ectopic ACTH syndrome (i.e. excess ACTH secretion from a carcinoma — most commonly a bronchial carcinoma).
**end**

**275.** b), c) and d).
**dy**

**276.** a), c) and d).
**ld**

**277.** a) Retained foreign body. Pulp space infection. Osteomyelitis.
b) X-ray examination. This showed rarefaction of the distal phalanx. There was no evidence of radiopaque foreign body. Culture fluid for organisms.
c) Incision and curettage of devitalized pulp and bone. Leave the wound open to drain. The wound should then heal spontaneously.
N.B.: Retained vegetable foreign bodies, e.g. wood, grass, thorns, etc. can pre-dispose to severe infections in the hand.
**hc**

**278.** Rest pain and intermittent claudication. Arterosclerosis with blockage of most of the arteries above and below the knee on both legs.
**pvd**

**279.** Twenty years ago this was a fairly common example of a tuberculous

abscess. It has been less frequent, indeed almost rare, in the past 10 years or so but is now being seen in the elderly and in those from overseas. Antituberculous drugs and local incision and drainage may be required.
gsd

280. b) and c).
ld

281. Pseudo diverticulum in right inguinal hernial sac.
ur

282. This is a benign melanotic naevus of which the size and degree of pigmentation may vary. Rapid growth, increase in pigmentation, ulceration or bleeding may indicate a change to malignancy. Examine lymphatic glands.
gsd

283. Marked blown up thigh veins due to varicose veins with blow outs may lead to thrombophlebitis. These should be treated by compression bandaging until the inflammatory response resolves.
pvd

284. Tumour of testis is the most likely diagnosis. Sometimes these patients may have pain and are suspected as having epididymitis but the redness and oedema in this is absent. Lymphangiography will give some ideas of the extent of the spread.
gsd

285. Ewing tumour in the upper end of the tibia at an advanced stage which has not responded to radiotherapy.
clo

286. a) Fired point blank.
chtr

287. 1. Old injury.  2. Viral

Infections.  3. Dry eye syndrome. This case is a Dry Eye Syndrome.
col

288. a) X-linked recessive
    b) 1 in 2
    c) Three CPKs in a laboratory with an obligate carrier range
    clge

289. a) This is hairy tongue — brought about by elongation of the filiform papillae.
    b) The aetiology is unknown but some cases follow a course of antibiotic therapy.
    c) The condition may be resistant to treatment of all kinds. In other cases it spontaneously regresses.
    om

290. Harrison.
    nd

291. The ulceration may be related to varicose veins or result from a previous deep vein thrombosis. About 60% are postphlebitic. Help may be gained from a good history, physical examination, presence of leg pulses, absence of sensation and medication used. About 70% have contact hypersensitivity. These cases are difficult to treat.
    pvd

292. The diagnosis is Keratoconus which is an overall thinning of the cornea.
    col

293. a) Acute purulent otitis media.
    b) *Streptococcus pneumoniae; Streptococcus viridans* and *Haemophilus influenzae.*
    ed

294. Paget's Disease.
    bd

295. Middle lobe benign enlarged prostate. Signs of outflow obstruction — dilated tortuous lower ureters and diverticulum on left.
ur

296. Right-sided diverticulum — Right ureter stretched over it.
ur

297. b). Benign paroxismal positional vertigo
ent

298. a) Bilateral cleft lip; pits on the lower lip
b) Van der Woude syndrome
c) Autosomal dominant
clge

299. a) Paralysis of the right side of the palate. Because of this the uvula moves up to the left when the patient says 'ah'.
b) A lower motor neurone lesion of the vagus nerve. (The vagus, like the facial nerve supply to the brow, has a bilateral upper motor neurone innervation, and the palate is not affected in a hemiplegia).
c) i) Lesions in the medulla — e.g. Wallenberg's lateral medullary syndrome, in which difficulty with swallowing is one of the most distressing features.
ii) Lesions in the region of the jugular foramen — e.g. a glomus jugulare tumour, nasopharyngeal carcinoma, carcinomatous or bacterial meningitis or a basilar aneurysm.
cln

300. a) Winging of the scapula.
b) Weakness of the serratus anterior due to damage to the long thoracic nerve. (Lesions of the accessory nerve also cause winging because the trapezius is weak, but in these patients the scapula is pulled downwards by the serratus anterior).
c) Neuralgic amyotrophy and trauma.
cln

301. a) Precocious puberty
b) Advanced
c) Congenital adrenal hyperplasia
end

302. This is a melanoma which fortunately for the patient was benign. A biopsy was inconclusive and therefore radical vulvectomy was carried out. A wide excision with hindsight would have been more appropriate treatment.
clgy

303. This lesion could easily be mistaken for an epithelioma. The rapid growth, volcanic-like appearance, and absence of lymphadenopathy suggest that it is a KERATOCANTHOMA (MOLLUSEUM SEBACEUM). (Often there is a KERATIN plug). Excision or curettage and cautering will clean the lesion up.
gsd

304. b). Erysipelas
ent

305. a) It could be a concomitant squint — in which case the patient would fixate with the left eye when the right is covered. In fact, the patient was unable to abduct the right eye when looking to that side because of a right sixth nerve palsy.
b) None.
c) "Idiopathic — ? vascular" and diabetes.
cln

**306.** a) This is the oral presentation of erythema multiformae. The involvement of the lower lip is common although this is a particularly severe example.

b) Target lesions may appear on the skin although the oral mucosa only may be involved.

c) Many precipitating factors have been described including drugs and attacks of facial herpes. However, most cases are apparently without a precipitating factor.

om

**307.** a) An atrial septal defect, premium type.

b) Below.

c) The defect involves the atrio-ventricular valves and the arrow points at a cleft in the anterior leaflet of the mitral valve.

cpa

**308.** b), c), d) and e).

ld

**309.** a) Tuberose sclerosis.

b) Adenoma sebaceum on chin. Shagreen patch on forehead.

c) 1 in 2.

d) Look for appropriate skin lesions — especially white macules under a Wood's lamp and do a CT scan to look for intracranial calcification if in doubt.

clge

**310.** a) Dystrophia myotonica.

b) Frontal baldness, ptosis, wasting of the temporalis muscles and a weak, expressionless face.

c) Cataracts, atrophy of the sternomastoids, weakness, a myotonic grip and gonadal atrophy.

d) Anaesthetic disasters due to impairment of cardio/respiratory function and — in the long term

— paralysis due to the muscular dystrophy.

cln

**311.** a) Myocardial infarction.

b) The first myocardial slice shows a regional type and the second a laminar type. The regional type illustrated shows infarction of the full width of the posterior left ventricular wall and posterior half of the interventricular septum in the region of the supply of the right coronary artery. The laminar type myocardial infarction involving the inner half of the left ventricular free wall and the left half of the interventricular septum is usually seen in hearts with severe atheroma of all the main coronary arteries, but may also occur in association with regional infarcts.

cpa

**312.** b), c) and e).

gem

**313.** Cholesterol

i) Atheroma

ii) Xanthoma

iii) Old abscesses and haematomas

iv) Lipid pneumonia

v) Cholesterolosis of gall bladder

sp

**314.** a), d) and e).

gem

**315.** This was a CIRSOID aneurysm which is a complicated arterio-venous fistula of the scalp vessels. There is a marked thrill and bruit if not thrombosed.

pvd

**316.** a) There is gross wasting in the first left dorsal interspace. There is also a suggestion of wasting and

272

of guttering on the right, and of wasting of the left hypothenar mass.

b) An ulnar neuropathy, syringomyelia and motor neurone disease.

c) If the wasting is generalised, the tendon reflexes are preserved and sensation is normal the patient probably has motor neurone disease. If the arm reflexes are absent and pain and temperature sensation are impaired in the upper limbs, he probably has syringomyelia. (Both conditions can cause fasciculation and a spastic paraplegia). If the wasting is confined to one hand, sparing much of the thenar mass, and the reflexes are intact but the sensation is impaired over the medial one and a half digits he probably has an ulnar neuropathy.

**cln**

317. It can occur with any condition associated with generalised oedema, cardiac disease, cirrhosis renal failure. In this case, the patient had a nephretic syndrome.
**clgy**

318. Yes to b) and c), d) and a) possibly.
**bd**

319. a) Bilateral Madelung's deformity.
b) Dyschondrosteosis.
c) Mild short stature; autosomal dominant.
**clge**

320. The farm worker had recently been carrying sacks of bone-meal on his shoulder. A smear of the fluid from a vesicle was found to contain the ANTHRAX bacillus.
**gsd**

321. a) Overwear of large thick soft lenses.
b) Chronic dry eye. Inflammatory lid reactions. Viral infection such as trachoma.
**col**

322. The right leg is swollen compared with the left. There is oedema of the vulva on the right side. Left labia majora is just visible. No obvious scars on the abdomen or the groin to suggest a surgical cause. The cause was obstruction of the lymphatics due to the parasitic worm Wuchereria bancrofti, transmitted by mosquitoes.
**clgy**

323. a) These small ulcers were due to a herpes infection which is occurring with increasing frequency. Soreness is a more common complaint than irritation.
b) Behçets Syndrome. In this case, the oral and vulval lesions were confirmed to be due to herpes infection.
**clgy**

324. a) Aschoff's node.
b) Rheumatic heart disease.
c) This is a granulomatous lesion that occurs in the stromal connective tissue. The fully developed Aschoff's node illustrated here consists of central fibrinoid material surrounded by histiocytes and scanty lymphocytes, plasma and giant cells. The characteristic histiocyte, or Anitschkow, cells are large with a slight basophilic cytoplasm. Their nuclei contains a central bar of chromatin from which fine strands radiate outwards. When cut in cross sections the nuclei may resemble "owl's eyes" and in longitudinal

273

sections caterpillars. The giant or Aschoff cells typically contain 3-4 centrally placed nuclei and are also of histiocytic origin.

**cpa**

325. a) An internuclear ophthalmoplegia. The patient is unable to adduct his left eye when looking to the right. The third nerve and medial rectus are evidently intact, for the eye adducts normally on convergence. The lesion lies in the left medial longitudinal bundle, which connects the pontine centre for conjugate gaze to the right (in the region of the sixth nerve nucleus) with the contralateral third nerve.
    b) The sign is most often seen in multiple sclerosis, when it is bilateral. It also occurs with ischaemic lesions, when it is commonly unilateral.

**cln**

326. a) Turner's syndrome.
    b) Oedema of hands and feet and hypoplastic nails as a neonate. Short stature, shield-like chest, cubitus valgus, primary amenorrhoea with streak gonads, coarctation of the aorta (15%) and keloid formation.
    c) Chromosome analysis shows a 45, X chromosome complement. Buccal smear analysis to look for Barr bodies is not adequate.

**clge**

327. a) Wasting of the buttocks.
    b) Inability to climb stairs, get out of deep armchairs and board buses — activities which require powerful hip extension.
    c) Hereditary disorders (muscular dystrophies). Inflammatory disorders (polymyositis). Endocrine disorders (e.g. Cushing's disease,

thyrotoxicosis, diabetes). Metabolic disorders (e.g. hypercalcaemia). Carcinoma.

**cln**

328. A popliteal aneurysm was leaking into the tissues. These aneurysms may be bilateral. In this case of unilateral aneurysm, a resection was performed and a graft inserted.

**pvd**

329. a) Carpal tunnel syndrome. This is the most likely cause of waking at night with paraesthesia in the median nerve distribution of the hand. Other conditions such as cervical spondylosis, spinal cord tumour, etc. can cause weakness and clumsiness and should be excluded by a thorough clinical examination with or without E.M.G. investigations.
    b) Because of the persisting symptoms and the signs of thenar muscle weakness and wasting, operative decompression is indicated.

**hc**

330. d). An osteoclastoma

**bd**

331. b). Possible post-traumatic colothorax

**chtr**

332. Haematoma of the vulva, which could be caused by a fall, post-operation or following childbirth and rarely following rape. The most common symptom in all cases is pain.

**clgy**

333. Usually seen in a diabetic with arterial disease. The vessels below the knee in this 54-year-old man were obliterated. He was a heavy smoker!!

**pvd**

**334.** a) A floppy valve or isolated mucoid (myxomatous) degeneration of the valve.
b) The mitral valve leaflets are stretched and ballooned giving a parachute-like appearance.
c) The stretching of the leaflets results from collagen degeneration associated with the presence of acid muco-polysaccharide and softening of the fibrosa layer of the valve cusp.
d) Mitral regurgitation may result from prolapsing of the valve. Rupture of a chordae tendineae may occur. Another complication is infective endocarditis. Rarely sudden death may occur.
cpa

**335.** EHLERS-DANLOS disease with loss of elasticity of the skin. This and MARFAN's syndrome are sometimes associated with dissecting aneurysms of the aorta.
pvd

**336.** a) Insulin lipodystrophy.
b) Vary the sites of injection. Use neutral pH insulins.
end

**337.** Primary generalised osteoarthritis is typified by involvement of *terminal* interphalangeal joints of the fingers in which Heberden's nodes can be seen on the dorsum of the joints.
clo

**338.** a) There is a large mass in the left upper zone.
b) Your immediate question is whether this is a benign or malignant tumour.
c) Make sure that an aortic aneurysm has been excluded by radiology. It is then safe to do a direct biopsy.

e) Surgical removal if there are no distant metastases. This was, in fact, a pleural fibroma.
resd

**339.** a) True
b) False
c) True
d) True
e) True
f) False
sp

**340.** a) Arachnodactyly.
b) Steinberg's thumb sign. When the thumb is adducted across the palm, the tip extends beyond the ulnar border.
c) Marfan syndrome; Homocystinuria; Frontometaphyseal dysplasia; Multiple mucosal neuroma syndrome; Beal's contractural arachnodactyly.
clge

**341.** a) No.
b) The commonest are oral contraceptives, phenothiazines, tricyclic antidepressants, methyl dopa, haloperidol and reserpine.
c) Primary hypothyroidism.
end

**342.** A carotid tumour or enlarged glands or aneurysm could be suspected. The long history and ultrasound supported the diagnosis of a carotid body tumour.
pvd

**343.** a) Hydrops Fetalis
b) Intrauterine infection; congenital nephrotic syndrome
nb

**344.** a) Behçet's syndrome
b) Hypopyon
c) Retinal vein occlusion
esd

**345.** Buerger's disease. Arteriography revealed the typical narrowing of the arteries below the knees in a tapering fashion. It responded to stoppage of smoking and sympathectomy.
**pvd**

**346.**
a) Vitiligo
b) Depigmentation; surrounding hyperpigmentation; approximately symmetrical distribution.
c) Autoimmune thyroid disease; Addison's disease; pernicious anaemia.
**end**

**347.**
a) Cavernous sinus thrombosis.
b) Staphylococcal infections of the face, nasal sinuses, mouth or pharynx.
c) Involvement of the contralateral sinus; damage to 2nd, 3rd, 4th, 5th and 6th cranial nerves; cerebral involvement with fits, hemiplegia and/or coma; septic pulmonary emboli.
d) Broad spectrum antibiotics given early, in large doses and for at least two months.
**cln**

**348.** Yes to b) and c).
**bd**

**349.** This is an effort thrombosis of the subclavian vein due to nipping of the vein between the clavicle and the first rib when the arm is extended upwards, Venography was confirmatory. Heparinisation was carried out and gradually the swelling diminished.
**pvd**

**350.** Tophus
a) True
b) True
c) False
d) True

e) True
f) True
g) True
**sp**

**351.** There was insufficient $O_2$ passing through the contact lens causing abnormal metabolism and a consequential neo-vascular response.
**col**

**352.**
a) Spasm of the facial muscles in a patient with tetanus.
b) Trismus; increased lumbar lordosis due to spasm of spinal muscles; spasm of the abdominal muscles without tenderness; limbs relatively supple between spasms; causative injury.
c) An adverse reaction to phenothiazines.
**cln**

**353.** b) and d).
**gem**

**354.**
a) Arachnodactyli or "spider fingers".
b) It could be either Marfan's syndrome, or Homocystinuria.
c) Dislocation of the lens (ectopia lentis). In Marfan's syndrome the lens usually dislocates supero-nasally, but inferiorly in homocystinuria.
**esd**

**355.** This is primary lymphoedema (tarda). The gradual occlusion of the few lymph channels occurred with the infection and the cellulitis progressed. Longterm antibiotic therapy is necessary.
**pvd**

**356.** d) and e).
**nb**

276

**357.** The fetal head with a fibroid polyp below it.
**clgy**

**358.** b), c) and e).
**hi**

**359.** a) A left facial palsy. Note the failure to bury the eyelashes, to bare the teeth fully and to contract the platysma on that side.
b) Ask the patient to wrinkle his brow.
c) In a lower motor neurone palsy (e.g. Bell's palsy) all the facial muscles on one side are paralysed. In an upper motor neurone palsy (e.g. a stroke) the muscles of the brow are spared because they are bilaterally innervated.
**cln**

**360.** a) Puberty gynaecomastia
b) No
c) Wait. It will probably resolve spontaneously.
**end**

**361.** a) Turner's syndrome
b) Neck webbing; low hairline; lymphoedema of hands
**nb**

**362.** b) and d).
**gem**

**363.** Yes to a) and b).
**bd**

**364.** Bipartite patella requires no treatment as a rule (it is *not* a fracture!) but in some cases where Chondromalacia is present excision of the fragment may be required.
**is**

**365.** a) Stellate cataract
b) Myotonic dystrophy
**esd**

**366.** b), c), d) and f).
**hi**

**367.** a) A left third nerve palsy.
b) In a pure third nerve palsy (e.g. due to an aneurysm on the posterior communicating artery) the left eye would be abducted because the 6th cranial nerve is intact. However, the marks on the patient's face suggest that the first division of the trigeminus is involved, in which case an aneurysm in the cavernous sinus is the most likely diagnosis. This would also damage the fourth and sixth nerves, leaving the eye in a neutral position.
When a third nerve palsy is due to compression the pupil is usually dilated because the parasympathetic pupillo-constrictor fibres are in a superficial, exposed position. However, a large aneurysm in the cavernous sinus may also damage sympathetic pupillo-dilator fibres in the trigeminal nerve, in which case the pupil would not dilate. In palsies due to 'metabolic' disorders (e.g. diabetes) the pupil is usually unaffected.
**cln**

**368.** Post-pregnancy amenorrhoea associated with lactation. If not pregnant, then galactorrhoea due to an excess of prolactin secretion and possible microadenoma of the pituitary. It can also be caused by drugs or excessive manipulation. A blood prolactin estimation, test of visual fields, X-ray of the pituitary fossa. Bromocriptine is an effective treatment for galactorrhoea and anovulation, if present.
**clgy**

**369.** a) There is a rusty-brown ring at the corneal periphery. It is

known as a Kayser-Fleischer ring, brought about by deposits of copper in Descamet's membrane.
b) Wilson's disease (hepatolenticular degeneration).
c) Sunflower cataract.
esd

370. c). d) possibly.
bd

371. Glomus tumour
a) from glomero-arteriovenous anastomosis
b) female preponderance
c) typically the terminal phalanx or nailbed
d) glomus cells, blood vessels and nerves
sp

372. 1) Right pelvic-ureteric obstruction with resulting hydronephrosis.
2) Left pelvic kidney.
ur

373. a) Tubercle, tumour and trauma. Tubercle is the least likely because it involves the disc spaces (causing narrowing) and adjacent vertebrae.
b) This was a fracture in one of the upper lumbar vertebrae (? $L_2$) — i.e. below the cord, which ends at $L_1$. Most of the lumbar roots will be in a relatively safe position at the sides of the canal, but the sacral roots of the cauda equina occupy a vulnerable central position. The likely findings are weakness of plantar flexion and loss of the ankle jerk (S1), loss of sensation on the back of the lower limbs (S1-5) and loss of bladder control (S2-4).
c) Urgent decompression.
cln

374. d) and e).
nb

375. a) Histiocytoma
b) (i) Lipid
(ii) Haemosiderin
c) No
d) Nil
sp

376. a) There are grey-brown branching angioid streaks which seem to arise from the margin of the optic disc. They are irregular in outline and lie beneath the retinal vessels. A macular scar is also present.
b) There may be a sudden loss of vision caused by haemorrhage from sub-retinal new vessels which develop in the angioid streaks. Involvement of the macula leads to scar formation and a central scotoma.
c) Grönblad-Strandberg syndrome, characterised by defects in the elastic tissues of the skin, eye and systemic arteries.
esd

377. a) Punched-out osteolytic lesions in the skull.
b) Multiple myelomatosis.
c) Recurrent respiratory and urinary infections due to depressed immunity against infection. The patient may lose height due to involvement of vertebrae and shrinking of the spinal column. There may also be evidence of hepatosplenomegaly, renal failure or even paraplegia due to spinal involvement.
d) Plasma-cell infiltration of bone marrow. Abnormal globulins in serum and in urine (Bence-Jones proteinuria). Hypercalcaemia. Widespread radiological involvement of bones.

e) Radiotherapy, steroids, melphalan, cyclophosphamide, interferon, antibiotics, plasmapheresis.
resd

**378.** b) and e).
nb

**379.** Amoebiasis cutis.
(i) Microscopic examination of fresh exudate from the wound for vegetative forms of Entamoebae histolytica.
(ii) Demonstrations in sections of amoebae showing erythrophagocytosis.
(iii) Serological tests including complement fixation, immunofluorescence, gel diffusion and haemaglutination.
(iv) Culture.
sp

**380.** This is an example of a very serious condition presenting as a sports injury. The patient has an osteosarcoma of the lower end of the femur. Failure to pay attention to persistent pain in cases of this type may lead to fatal delay before proper treatment is given.
is

**381.** Yes to c). Possibly b).
bd

**382.** a) Anophthalmia
b) Patau's syndrome
nb

**383.** Peri-oral rhagades from congenital syphilis.
ve

**384.** a) Narrowing of a disc space was followed by destruction of adjacent vertebral bodies due to a tuberculous paravertebral abscess (Pott's disease). The abscess shadow is well seen.
b) A needle, lying within the abscess cavity, is used to aspirate pus.
c) Vague undiagnosed backache for the previous two years.
d) Aspirated pus revealed acid-fast bacilli, and culture showed tubercle bacilli.
e) Antituberculous chemotherapy for 18 months to 2 years, with bed rest, and measures to make sure that final cure is achieved with a good postural result.
resd

**385.** b), c) and e).
nb

**386.** a) Subungual fibroma.
b) Tuberous Sclerosis (Bourneville's disease).
c) Glistening, mulberry-like astrocytomas which involve the optic disc and retina.
esd

**387.** a) Enlargement of the $^5/_6$ cervical intervertebral foramen. (Note difference in shape and narrowing of adjacent pedicles).
b) A 'dumbbell' neurofibroma, partly inside and partly outside the spinal canal.
c) (i) A spastic paraplegia due to compression of the cord.
(ii) A lower cervical radiculopathy (eg $C_6$ — weakness of biceps, loss of supinator jerk and impaired sensation over thumb and index, of $C_7$ — weakness of triceps, loss of triceps jerk and impaired sensation over middle finger).
(iii) (possibly) cutaneous lesions of neurofibromatosis.
cln

279

**388.** a) Absence of frontal cortex; fusion of lateral ventricles
b) Holeprosencephaly
**nb**

**389.** Lichen planus
**ve**

**390.** Osteoid osteoma. A benign tumour causing intense pain.
**clo**

**391.** a) Scabies
b) Herpes simplex; accidental vaccinia
**ve**

**392.** a) A cataract is present, the opacity in the centre of the lens having the appearance of an "oil drop"
b) Galactosaemia.
**esd**

**393.** a) Neuropathic chest.
b) Anything causing prenatal weakness of the thoracic muscles — e.g. Lejeune's.
**nb**

**394.** a) The writing is tremulous, but the letters are of a reasonable size and do not become smaller. These things suggest that the patient has an essential tremor, not Parkinson's disease.
b) An increase in the tremor when the limb is in use (a Parkinsonian tremor would usually diminish), a decrease after drinking alcohol, and a positive family history.
c) Propranolol.
**cln**

**395.** The patient has secondary syphilis.
a) Darkfield microscopy for Treponema pallidum. Material is obtained by lymph gland aspiration or from skin lesion scrapings.
c) Serological tests for syphilis,

invariably positive in the secondary stage.
**ve**

**396.** a) Erb's palsy
b) Neck hyperextension
c) $C_3$, $C_4$ and $C_5$.
**nb**

**397.** The woman was found to have gonorrhoea complicated by pelvic inflammation and bacteraemia. The early stages of gonococcal infection in women are usually asymptomatic and hence the presence of infection may only become evident when metastatic or other complications occur.
**ve**

**398.** b), c) and d).
**nb**

**399.** a) Corneal nebulae from previous interstitial keratitis.
b) Congenital syphilis.
**ve**

**400.** Fibrocystic disease of the breast.
a) True
b) False
c) False
d) False
e) True
f) True
**sp**